Surrendering
TO THE Call

Also by Marilee J. Bresciani

Forthcoming Books:
The Foundation is Love

Empowering Leaders out of the Politics of Decision-Making

Other Books:
Bresciani, M.J. (2011). *Rushing to yoga.* Bloomington, Indiana: Balboa Press.

Bresciani, M.J., Gardner, M.M., Hickmott, J. (2009). *Demonstrating student success.* Sterling, VA: Stylus Publishing.

Bresciani, M.J., Gardner, M.M., Hickmott, J. (Eds.). (2009). Case studies in assessing student success. *New Directions for Student Services, 127.* Boston, MA: Jossey Bass.

Bresciani, M.J. (ed.) (2007). *Good practice case studies for assessing general education.* Boston, MA: Jossey Bass.

Bresciani, M.J. (2006). *Outcomes-based academic and co-curricular program review.* Sterling, VA: Stylus Publishing.

Bresciani, M.J., Zelna, C. L., & Anderson, J.A. (2004). *Techniques for assessing student learning and development.* Washington D.C.: NASPA.

For more information, see
http://www.rushingtoyoga.org

Surrendering
TO THE Call

The Journey to Authenticity

MARILEE J. BRESCIANI, PH.D

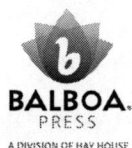

BALBOA.
PRESS
A DIVISION OF HAY HOUSE

Balboa Press books may be ordered through booksellers or by contacting:

Balboa Press
A Division of Hay House
1663 Liberty Drive
Bloomington, IN 47403
www.balboapress.com
1-(877) 407-4847

Because of the dynamic nature of the Internet, any web addresses or links contained in this book may have changed since publication and may no longer be valid. The views expressed in this work are solely those of the author and do not necessarily reflect the views of the publisher, and the publisher hereby disclaims any responsibility for them.

The author of this book does not dispense medical advice or prescribe the use of any technique as a form of treatment for physical, emotional, or medical problems without the advice of a physician, either directly or indirectly. The intent of the author is only to offer information of a general nature to help you in your quest for emotional and spiritual well-being. In the event you use any of the information in this book for yourself, which is your constitutional right, the author and the publisher assume no responsibility for your actions.

Any people depicted in stock imagery provided by Thinkstock are models, and such images are being used for illustrative purposes only.
Certain stock imagery © Thinkstock.

ISBN: 978-1-4525-4586-8 (e)
ISBN: 978-1-4525-4585-1 (sc)
ISBN: 978-1-4525-4587-5 (hc)

Library of Congress Control Number: 2012902344

Printed in the United States of America

Balboa Press rev. date: 2/28/2012

This book is dedicated to all those whom I love; all my teachers and students. I am so grateful for your presence in my life. Thank you for providing me the space to be all I am and all I am not.

"I used to think that becoming authentic took a lot of work. I didn't realize that the work was simply about making a choice; choosing to surrender to awakening one moment at a time."

-Marilee J. Bresciani, Ph.D.

CONTENTS

LIST OF ILLUSTRATIONS

The artworks featured on the cover and on the back were photographed by Jamie Gallant at his and his wife's home. I am so grateful to Jamie for contributing his time and talent. More of Jamie's photography can be found at www.THEcaskandbarrel.com

ACKNOWLEDGMENTS

I wish to acknowledge with deep gratitude the following beautiful souls for the role they played in the co-creation of this book. Thank you for all you have taught me. I am truly grateful!

Thank you Karl, Cyd, Ralph, Lauren, Elsa, Marva, Penny, Kevin, Barbara, Lori, Dani, Amorah, Adrian, Laura Lee, David, Gary, Dan, Cathy, Danny, Jan, Mike, Michael, Elizabeth, Cynthia, George, Jessica, Shaila, Baron, Philip, Ty, Kendra, Dean, Machala, Ixchel, Ruben, Andrea, Reo, John, Robert, Audrey, John, Christina, Fred, Caren, Sara, Tricia, Jamie, Carol, Gavin, Chris, Joshua, Scott, Ron, Irina, and Dad and Mom (although I hope you never read this; you will freak).

PREFACE

Mark Nepo [1]writes that "facing ourselves, uncovering the meaning in our hard experiences, the entire work of the consciousness speaks to a process by which we sculpt away the excess, all that we are not; finding and releasing the gesture of soul that is already waiting, complete, within us. Self-actualization is this process applied to our life on Earth."

The point that I understand Mark Nepo is making is that the journey to authenticity, the journey to surrendering to our individual call to be authentic is a journey of removing the excess from our lives. I understand from him that the only way we can discover that which is excess in our lives is through really living our lives. I mean *really* living our lives and discovering that which we are not by discovering that which we are and are becoming through lived experiences.

For example, I am not who I am or who I am becoming in my mind. For in my mind – the made up reality - I am a Princess, a scholar, a writer, a musician, an artist, an athlete, a goddess, a pain-in-the-ass employee, a demanding teacher, a daughter who lives too far away from her parents, and a friend who is not one you call upon if you want sympathy. However, these labels are more the roles or perceptions that have come to *be* in my life; they are the hats I put on and take off. None of those descriptors *is* authentically me at all. In my lived experiences however, I play all of those roles and more. However, through my lived experiences, I know more of what I am not. I am not a survivor. I am not a victim. I am not a Princess, a goddess, an artist, an athlete, or a scholar. In living, I am sculpting away the excess of what the mind

---

1   Mark Nepo, The Book of Awakening: Having the Life you Want by Being Present to the Life you Have.

brings to roles that I experience. In sculpting away the excess, it makes room for surrendering, surrendering to the call of my authenticity. In my authenticity, my soul is released and here is where joy, peace, and love are made present in the day-to-day. In surrendering to my authenticity, the roles fall away and what is left is the pureness of the soul and its expression. The soul and the expression of it never waivers, regardless of the role or the life situation in which it finds itself. Perhaps, another example taken from my personal journal may be helpful.

Last night, I was with some of my dear friends in a vacant old home. The home was painted white and there were no furnishings at all. I had no idea why I was there. We were gathered in the kitchen and I felt a bit "out of body". I was not even sure how I had gotten there let alone when I had arrived.

One of my friends was in the living room by herself. The rest of us were chatting about something in the kitchen but I really had no idea what we were even talking about. The friend who was in the living room let out a terrifying scream so we rushed to the entrance of where the kitchen greeted the living room to see what had happened. I saw her horrified expression across the living room; she literally appeared to be scared stiff, so I called out to her. When she didn't respond, I moved toward her. As I moved toward her, I felt a large energy force in the middle of the room; the force was occupying a large portion of the room. I was not afraid however; I felt that the energy was extremely dense, extremely powerful. I couldn't move through it. I had to move around it in order to get to her. I asked her to calm down, to not fear the energy force but to move slowly around it back toward my other friends who were waiting, mouths opened wide but seemingly less horrified, in the entrance way to the kitchen.

As I made my way to where my friend had been standing and as she made her way to the entrance to the room where my friends stood, I turned to face the energy force. As I turned to look upon it, it began to rush toward me. I could feel that it wanted to attack me but I had no idea why.

I held up my hand in front of my face as if to say, "Don't even try it, 'cause you don't want to mess with me." But to my great surprise, my hand didn't hold the attacking force. Instead, the force grabbed me by both of my arms, twirled me around, and threw me down onto my back. I landed hard onto the floor, all of the air escaping from my body. As I began to regain my ability to breathe again, the force let go of my arms, twirled me around on my back and then grabbed me by the legs and began to swing me around the room as if I was nothing more than a rag doll.

I was so shocked that I couldn't stop the force from swinging me around. I couldn't' see it but I felt it. I was so annoyed and becoming more anxious because I had no idea why all this was happening. I tried to communicate with it, reason with it, but nothing worked. It just kept swinging me round and round in circles. I began to try to anticipate what would happen next and as I saw what was coming, I felt a bit of panic.

The force was swinging me out wider and wider; it was as if its arms were getting longer and the circumference of the swing was getting wider. Soon, my head would crash into the wall. Just as my head was about to swing into the wall, I realized that I could keep myself from getting hurt. So, with one thought, I made the wall disappear, but just the portion where my head would have made contact with the wall.

"This is cool," I thought to myself. I can make the wall disappear so I don't get hurt while this force is swinging me around but I can't get it to stop swinging me around. I don't know how to communicate with it, or reason with it. I have no idea why it attacked me and I have no idea how to make it stop. But I can make sure I don't get hurt while it is whirling me around. That is pretty cool. Once I realized that the whirling crazed force of energy could not hurt me, even though I could not stop it, or reason with it, or manage it, or understand what was happening and why, I realized that I was fully occupying my body and that I was at peace. And then, I awoke.

I was now awake. I had been dreaming. I was once again, feeling a bit out of body. I rolled over and looked at my Love. He didn't seem to be bothered by my nightmare at all; he seemed to be peacefully resting on his back. I was so shocked to find myself in bed with him, to discover that I had not already awakened for I thought I had. For in the dream that I had apparently just had, a part of the dream was waking with Karl and then my hurrying to get my suitcase packed for the trip back to San Diego, boarding the plane, getting off the plane and then meeting my friends who were in the white roomed house. Until this moment, the point that I saw him lying next to me, I had no idea that

I had actually been dreaming. I thought the encounter with the force of energy was real.

I poked Karl and awakened him.

"Karl, am I awake? Or am I dreaming?"

Karl had been lying peacefully on his back. In response to my persistent poking, he opened one eye and looked at me, he smiled his half smile – the one that warms my heart and melts my soul – and then he closed his eye again.

I poked him again.

"Karl, seriously, am I awake or am I dreaming?"

He responded with a very loud and very long fart. But I was still not convinced I was not dreaming. For in the dream that I had just had where I thought I was awake; in the dream I had just had where I had dreamt waking up with him in this exact bed and this exact moment, he had also farted. So this behavior was not convincing me at all that I was awake. I thought that I still could be dreaming.

"Kaaarrrllll", I moaned, this time pushing his shoulders, moving his upper body back and forth on the bed. He half smiled again and put his arm out, folding me into him kissing my forehead. The sensation of his loving touch and kiss moved through my body and I realized in that moment, that I was no longer dreaming. I thanked him for helping me understand that I was now awake or at least feeling awake.

"I had a really weird dream." I said to him, my voice a little muffled, for my head was buried in his side. I didn't mind that my voice was incoherent; I liked being there.

Hearing my muffled voice, he released his loving hold on me so I could move away from him to tell him about the dream in detail.

"That is a weird one." He slowly and softly responded when I finished telling him about it. "Good luck figuring out what that one means," he joked with me but I didn't laugh.

I always laugh at his jokes. I think he is the funniest man in the world. But this time, I didn't laugh. Feeling my tension, Karl gave me a tight squeeze and he spoke again.

"Maybe this one doesn't mean anything. Maybe it was just a bad dream."

As I returned his tight squeeze with a kiss and a smile, I laid back down by his side and closed my eyes. I prayed for an interpretation. I prayed to the Holy Spirit asking for help in understanding this most powerful message. Later that morning, after two cups of Karl's fabulous French press coffee, after packing my bag for San Diego, and after the woman who was seated next to me on the plane flight home accidentally kicked me for the third time in the shin, I pulled out my journal to record the dream and as I recorded the dream, the meaning came.

Life's experiences come at you whether you think you can control them or not. They come at you sometimes in attack and sometimes in exuberant joy. Sometimes, life experiences knock you on your back and other times they have you swinging around for joy or swinging around in anxiety, anticipating that you will be flung into a wall and broken into pieces, far too many pieces to ever hope of being put back together again.

Surrendering is letting go of the belief that I can control what life tosses my way. Surrendering is letting go of the belief that I can manage what life throws at me. Sometimes, no amount of reasoning, communication, or understanding changes anything I experience. Surrendering means letting go of managing all that is around me. In letting go of managing, I let go of the excess of that which is not mine to tend to and thus, that which is not me; that which does not resonate with my authenticity.

Surrendering is accepting. Acceptance is the realization that I can choose to be deeply wounded by the experiences of life or I can choose to recognize that obstacles causing permanent damage can be removed, buffered, or rendered non-existent. That which causes pain can be let go. That which distracts me from my authentic expression of joy, love, and peace can be let go.

Nothing in life is controllable. Acceptance of that is not passive; it involves a deep awareness of what I know and what I don't know, what I feel and what I don't feel, and what I see and what I don't see. Acceptance involves, as Mark Nepo describes, living away the excess so that the soul can return to its authenticity of love, joy, and peace. Surrendering is accepting who I am and who I am not and being open to whom I am becoming. However, do I hear the call to become authentic? And if I hear it, will I surrender to that call? Will I have the courage to face all that I am not to discover all that I am and am becoming?

I offer this book, filled with dramatized stories of conversations and experiences with friends and family members, to encourage you in your journey of removing the excess of who you think you are or who you have been told to become in order to return to your soul authenticity. The names have been changed to protect the identities of my teachers and the stories have been exaggerated to make the lessons learned clearer. I pray that these stories bring you courage and peace to move further into your own personal journey of authentic joy and love. The stories have helped me shed a little more of whom I am not, in order to surrender to the call of becoming who I am.

Namaste,

Marilee

INTRODUCTION

"You don't like it?" I asked with a mix of disappointment and anxiety, waiting to hear the answer from my spiritual mentor and priceless friend.

"It's not that I don't like it..." she hesitated. I could feel her compassion and love through my cell phone, yet my anxiety grew, waiting breathlessly for her answer. "It's just that it doesn't seem to be resonating at the level where you are in this moment."

I sighed a sigh of great relief as I burst into laughter.

"Thank you Dharma." I responded. "Thank you for saying that. No, it does not represent where I am today. It represents my journey getting here. "

She did not respond to my defensive declaration. So, in order to alleviate the pain of the silence I felt, I asked a stupid question...

"Did ya at least think it was funny?"

I could feel her patient and Buddha-like smile radiate through my tiny mobile phone.

"Yes Marilee, it was funny. However, was humor more valuable than resonating at your highest level?"

Well that was a damn good question, I thought to myself and I knew I couldn't lie to her.

"Well, yes, actually, I wanted it to be funny. I wanted it to appeal to an audience that may not typically be looking for spiritual enlightenment. You know, sort of how I met you. I wasn't looking for an awakening. You just happened to present an opportunity of one to me. I wanted to provide an opportunity for folks to begin to question – through humor – surprising them with an opportunity to awaken when they weren't even looking."

Again, I could feel her love pour over the airwaves and into my body. She was pure beauty, pure love, pure wisdom, and I was so grateful to have her in my life.

"I understand Marilee," she started softly. "Now, however, it is time for us to hear your words resonating at the level where you now appear." Her voice was soft and soothing, yet her message was challenging and filled with the kind of truth that cuts to your core; the kind of truth that can't be ignored.

"Well that message won't be very funny." I said with great sincerity and seriousness, which to my surprise caused her to laugh her hearty laugh that I so loved to hear.

"Well," she responded with continued compassion. "You'll figure it out."

With that, I hung up the phone. As I looked down to see how much battery power I had left, I realized that I had just lost cell phone reception completely. It was nearing the end of the day and I was driving down an icy snow-packed road, headed from the city into the mountains for a weekend meditation retreat – not a formal one, just one that I would create on my own – one that I decided I needed to experience.

This is not the slightest bit ironic, I thought. I had just ended a phone call that held a challenging message from a goddess and then I lost contact with civilization, as I know it. Apparently, it was time for another wake-up call.

As I drove into the starlit, stark cold night, alone in my Jeep with snow and ice on the roads and no ability to call anyone, I began to laugh aloud at the thought of it all. The roads were deserted, no car lights in site, no road lights in site, no radio reception, no phone reception, pure isolation and I could feel the presence of holiness; the holiness was not mine.

Hell no, so not mine. The presence of holiness came from the absence; the absence of sound, the absence of light, the absence of distraction, the absence of clarity.

"How do I write the next book without being funny?" [2] I said aloud in my empty Jeep. "Who wants to read something that isn't funny anyway?"

In the moment shortly after my proclamation, I hit a patch of ice. A four-wheel drive vehicle, even the noblest of all 4-wheel drive vehicles - Jeep Wranglers - doesn't do much for you when you aren't paying attention to how to use it. Before I could really fully remember how to pull myself out of a skid, I realized that I really didn't know how to pull myself out of a skid on the narrow road that hugged the side of the mountain. In a word, I thought I was pretty much "fucked."

In the moment that I found myself completely out of control, fish-tailing all over the road and wondering whether I would still be on the road as it curved sharply right to wind its way around the mountain, I thought about panicking. I remembered I had no cell phone access and I remembered that it had been a long time since I practiced pulling out of black ice skids. I had lived in the south far too long. So, panicking seemed to be a good idea. Instead, however, the words of Reyal[3] and thousands of others spoken before him came echoing to my mind. SURRENDER! And so I did.

By surrender, I don't mean I let go of the wheel and closed my eyes, but I think I did absolutely nothing. And as such, in the next moment, I was driving down the road, in full control of my vehicle, in my lane, still very much on the road and driving like nothing had ever happened.

"AWESOME!" I screamed at the top of my lungs. "That was awesome!" I screamed out again and then I broke into praises of gratitude for the lesson and the direction that had come so quickly in a such a brief moment on a cold, dark, isolated evening on this road where I was going no where in particular except somewhere to find a place to retreat.

This book is about my journey of surrendering to a call that I didn't know was mine, to a dream that I wasn't sure was just my mind's

---

2   The follow-up book to "Rushing to Yoga" by Balboa Press (2011).
3   Bresciani, M.J. (2011). *Rushing to Yoga*. Bloomington, IN: Balboa Press.

creation, and to a life I had no idea how to live. Similar to the journey that led me to this place, the journey of surrendering happened in the day-to-day, moment-by-moments of life. While I sought spiritual retreats to enlighten me and to strengthen me, they were all completed amidst the work that I did to earn my living, the work that I love to do and the work that "pays the bills."

I offer this journey to you, the reader, in the hopes that it will inspire you and cause you to question who you are and who you are becoming and whether you are responding to your own call to live a life in authenticity. I offer it to you in the hopes that you will explore what surrender means to you and that you will share the lessons you learned with another.

I teach what I need to learn. You provide me the opportunity to learn at a deeper level; you provide me with the opportunity to practice what I am learning and practice who I am becoming. And as such, I am forever grateful to you.

Namaste,

Marilee

CHAPTER ONE

Larger than Life Lori

"Can you tell me that again Lori?" I needed to hear it again. I couldn't believe my ears.

"If you don't begin making some different choices, about how you live your life immediately, you are going to be very, very, very sick."

Lori, [4]the woman who one of my dear friend's told me I just <u>had</u> to meet, was sitting across the beer stained table right in front of me. I paused a moment as her words landed in my mind. I looked around the Mexican bar. This was the weirdest place to get an astrology reading, a Mexican bar that reeked of the odors from the New Year's Eve party the night before. When I had first walked into the place, I was concerned about sitting anywhere, let alone stepping onto the floor; it had not yet been cleaned this New Year's Day morning. Nonetheless, here I was sitting across from larger than life Lori listening to her read my astrological chart.

Lori, as I think anyone who met her would describe her, is larger than life. She has a powerful personality and way of being about her. She is confident in her ability to read and interpret astrological charts and she is simply confident about who she is. A stout African-American woman and self-proclaimed bitch (seriously, she loves to be called a

---

bitch and purposefully invited me to do so), was delivering me an astrological reading I found based on love and nothing more. The words she just spoke however, were landing a little hard on my ears and in my mind.

"How sick?" I asked Lori as I leaned forward in my sticky chair, still too concerned to place my elbows on the table where she had the chart laid out in front of me.

"Very, very, very sick," she responded with no hesitation, no break in her eye contact with me, and with the same firmness in which she first announced this declaration.

"Like cancer sick?" I asked further, placing my left hand on my abdomen wondering if the surgery that I had just cancelled to have my ovaries removed was a wise decision or simply one made out of fear.

At this point, she looked down at the chart again, not in question of her interpretation but as if to read it in a way that she was actually reading the words verbatim.

"Very, very, very sick," she said again, with the matching affirmation of the previous two statements.

I felt my eyes begin to sting with tears or perhaps it was the smoke hanging from the night before that was stinging my eyes. I wasn't sure and in this moment, I didn't think it really mattered.

"Look Marilee, you have choices to make, right here, right now, right in this moment and in the moments that lie in front of you. What choices are you going to make?"

"I am sure as hell going to make different ones, but how and what? I have no idea. Anything in there to help me with that?" I was serious about what was coming out of my mouth.

She smiled now and let out a laugh that matched my own laugh's resonance and volume. The sound of it comforted my heart and I felt immediately at peace. *Yes,* I thought to myself, *Lori is larger than life for she is life.*

"You know that is not what this session is about. I am about empowering you to empower yourself. My role here is to prod and to coach you into your greatness, not tell you what to do." She continued to laugh heartily as giggling just was not in her repertoire.

Grateful for her honesty, I began to share the dreams I was having over the last 6 months; dreams that were clear in their colorful presentations in my mind, dreams that were as real as my waking life, and dreams that were powerful in stirring emotions deep within me. Yet as powerful as these dreams were, I was not yet clear in the messages they were trying to convey.

"I think the dreams have something to do with me facilitating myself and others in choosing to walk a daily life that is truly born out of love. But I don't know how to do that and I don't know what it looks like." Lori's response surprised me as she laughed heartily again. *I had no idea I was so amusing.* "I am serious Lori. Can you offer any guidance here?"

As Lori's loving laughter died down, she shared with me a great many strategies for opening myself so that I could better listen to the Holy Spirit's (what I call my God's) [5]prodding. She reminded me how powerful dreams are as a communication tool and reminded me to record my dreams as soon as I woke from them. She encouraged me not to try to figure them out. Rather, I was to write them down and their interpretation would come from the Holy Spirit when it was time.

Lori's advice was great advice and it was reaffirmed by a visit I made to my former meditation teacher and psychic medium, Chris, about a month after this conversation with Lori. The only challenge that remained which neither Lori or Chris could help me with was my own impatience for getting the interpretations to these dreams. I wanted the answers and I wanted them now. So, I pressed Lori further.

"Thanks Lori, this really is helpful but you mentioned the urgency of my needing to make changes and quite frankly, I feel that urgency;

---

5   An explanation of what God is and what the Holy Spirit is to me are found in a later chapter. For now, to me as I practice, God, the Holy Spirit, the Creator, my Source Power, the All Knowing One, and the Universe are used interchangeably. To me, they are the same names for the One that encompasses all that we know and do not know; the true Source of life, soul, spirit, intelligence, humor, peace, joy, love, and all other energy and matter seen and unseen.

I feel it in every cell of my being. That is why I am here. I mean, I feel illness in my body. I also feel restlessness, impatience, and aggravation. I know that the way I have been living is not the way I am to be living and I don't know how to live differently. I really need practical strategies. Is there anything in there to help me with that?"

I expected Lori to laugh again, but she didn't. Instead she leaned back on the wicker chair in which she was seated, slid the chart away from her, and closed her eyes.

In this moment, all I could think about quite frankly, was that I was grateful that I was not paying her by the hour because I was sure she was about ready to take a nap or go into deep meditation. Actually, I wasn't sure what she was doing or what she was going to do, but I knew whatever it was, it was going to be a while before I heard from her again. So, I flipped open my journal and began to write a few notes, when I saw that I had recorded the dream I had the night before. *How odd, I forgot I had recorded that.*

Looking back up at Lori to affirm that she was indeed in a state that would provide me with some reading time, I read from my journal to myself while Lori did whatever she was doing.

As I laid my head to sleep last night, I distinctly remember thinking, for some odd reason, that should I die before I wake, I will be fine. I was thinking that I felt so at peace. It was odd to feel so at peace on New Year's Eve, un-partnered yet in the loving company of glorious friends that I adored. And while I knew that my soul's journey had not been made complete this time around (whatever that really means anyway), I was at peace with knowing I was incomplete and I was loved anyway. It was a cool feeling. So I dreamt that I died. I really thought I died. I mean, in my dream state, I died. Dying was very peaceful.

In my dream, as I died, I felt my body begin to twirl like a cyclone but instead of a cyclone swirling up everything around it, I felt my bodies' cells begin to dissipate. It looked and felt more like Kool-Aid crystals that you stir ferociously in a glass of water, yet they refused to dissolve. I felt my cells pull apart in some sort of Kool-Aid like vortex and it was all very peaceful. I felt no pain. I felt only peace. Then I heard a voice, calling me to go back, to go back to body. So all of a sudden, the Kool-Aid crystals were gone and there I was, back in a body back on earth, living a journey, repeating lessons already learned, feeling frustrations, pain, and anger, sorrow and joy, disappointment and confusion. All I could think of was 'not again'. I gotta do this again. I gotta learn all these lessons again. This sucks. I want to live and I want to learn it this time around. I don't want to repeat lessons that I already learned, lessons that I already know. I want to learn new lessons. I don't want to die if it means I have to repeat this same life again to learn the same lessons again and to discover all that I know and don't know again. No way Jose, I mean Jesus, or God...no way, no thank you. And then...I awoke.

As I finished reading the passage from my journal, I felt a presence; I felt eyes upon me. So I looked up. It was Lori. I had gotten so pulled into reading my journal that I had forgotten where I was. I had forgotten that Lori was still there. She was smiling. I smiled back. It was a cool smiling connection. A rainbow may have even erupted between the smiles or one may have emerged out of them, but I couldn't see it because the bar was so dark, even though the sun was shining outside, even though it was early afternoon.

"Well?" she smiled brighter. It was a knowing smile. And I realized again, that I was in the presence of something larger than life, I was in the presence of love.

"I dreamt that I died last night." Her smile didn't break so I continued to explain to her what I had written in my journal. She listened and then she spoke.

"Write Marilee. Write. Quit dumbing down the messages that are being given to you. Quit being afraid of what others will think as they read them. Write, act, produce, return to the creative being that you have been stifling and who so desperately wants to assist in your journey here. Don't ignore what your heart speaks. Play, sing, paint, laugh heartedly, and smile at everyone you meet. Be joy. Be love. Quit critiquing yourself. Love yourself and then allow that love to heal. Be the magic you were created to be."

Tears of joy began streaming down my face as I heard Lori's words of encouragement. They felt like much more than words of encouragement to me as they resonated fully within my heart. My heart felt like it wanted to burst out of my chest in song and praise to the Universe, to the Creator, to God my Father and to the Holy Spirit my guide.

My tears mixed with my laughter as I sang praises of thanks to Lori and to the Universe for Lori and to the sticky beer-stained table and to the dark bar room smoky stinky air. I had died last night. It wasn't a dream after all. And today was the beginning of my life anew. Today was the first day for new lessons; today was the first day of letting go of the old self and inviting in the new. Today was truly New Year's Day.

Lori equipped me with mantras, readings, affirmations, and assignments. I had invited her to be my coach, to facilitate my new decision-making. Illness no longer had its grip on my body. It was time to release the creative heart spirit within and do so without judgment. And so off I went reciting my first affirmation from Lori. *I am a happy child. My smile and my laughter heal. I am a happy child. Time to heal.*

CHAPTER TWO

Jesus was in My Jeep

"Well, you got a lot of advice today Marilee. How are you feeling?" Carlos, asked me gently as I shuffled my feet in the warm sand of Coronado beach. It felt good to be walking along the ocean in the glorious February sun particularly after having been in a seminar all morning long. I didn't want to really answer Carlos' question, but at the same time, I felt that perhaps in answering it, I would feel a release that I needed to feel.

"I feel like shit. I mean I know everyone was trying to show up in love but honestly, I feel beat up. I feel worn out. I feel like shit." I didn't even look up at him as I spoke. I kept my eyes on my red painted toenails melting into the sand with each slow step I took.

I love having my toes in the sand. I love pedicures and I love red nail polish.

Carlos laughed softly and I could feel his love and peace radiate out toward me. I looked up at him as he laughed. He didn't even have to put his arm around me; he didn't have to look into my eyes. I could still feel his love even though he was also looking down at the sand between his toes.

Carlos had the kind of love that radiated far beyond his body. I often thought that hanging out with Carlos had to be a lot like hanging out with Jesus - the great teacher of how to live a loving life and how to simply be Love. Carlos was pure beauty and peace. I smiled as he was also clearly amused by his toes in the sand as well, for he spoke what we were both thinking (without the reference to pedicures and red polished toes). "I love the feel of my toes in the warm sand."

We kept walking in silence and then Carlos said, "You practiced well this morning Marilee."

I stopped in my tracks, shaken from my admiration of my red nail polish clashing against the beige, black, and gold grains of sand. I looked up at Carlos in shock.

"I practiced well? I practiced well? Carlos, I showed up in confusion, utter and complete confusion. How was *that* practicing well?"

Carlos smiled his gentle smile, spoke in his gentle voice and said, "You practiced what ACIM[6] speaks of as showing up in complete defenselessness. You showed up in open inquiry. You did well." With that, he gracefully continued walking down the beach.

As Carlos moved on, I was still standing in shock. I had no idea what he was talking about. I turned to the ocean and then looked up at the sky searching for some sign of clarity. Nothing came; I had no clue what he was talking about. So I turned quickly and ran to catch up with him even though running wasn't necessary. He hadn't gotten that far; he was still in his meditative stroll state.

"Carlos, I am sorry to bother you again but I don't understand what you are saying. Can you please help me understand?"

Carlos stopped walking and looked at me. He was skilled at mindfulness and I rarely saw him do two things at once. I so admired him and I took a deep breath not because I was in awe of him but because I was always so positively impacted by his love-filled looks.

Carlos was looking at me but this time, he was not smiling.

"As you asked questions about how to apply today's lessons to a specific situation in your life, you did not become defensive as people gave you various suggestions for how to do things differently. You simply acknowledged what you were hearing and then asked more questions.

---

6   A Course in Miracles – www.acim.org

It was clear you didn't understand how to apply the suggested advice to your situation but you didn't become defensive. You continued to show up in defenselessness. As such, it often feels like attack."

"It did feel like attack. It felt like a lot of judgment too and I felt very misunderstood." I hastily replied.

He didn't respond. So I added more for good measure.

"I don't want to practice defenselessness anymore." I wanted to laugh at the sound of what my ears just heard come out of my mouth but then I realized that I meant those words. I wasn't joking. I genuinely felt those words. So, I didn't laugh. And neither did Carlos.

With that declarative statement, Carlos responded with a question.

"In choosing to no longer practice that which you desire to learn, how do you expect to learn it?"

Now, that was funny. So, I laughed aloud, so heartily that the sea gulls who were searching for food about 25 yards in front of us took off in flight in fear. Or at least that is how I saw it.

"That's a damn good point Carlos. Thank you for *that* reminder." That was another thing I loved about Carlos. I felt that I could say anything around him and not be judged. *I wonder if that is how the Disciples felt around Jesus.*

We walked in silence to the point of the beach where we were compelled to turn around, because it was the part of the beach that the Navy owned and civilians were not allowed to walk there. I thought we would simply walk back to the Jeep and head back to the seminar location from where Carlos and I had car pooled to the beach for my current clarity walk but Carlos had a better idea; a much better idea.

"Let's go check out possible locations for your photographer to shoot the cover of your book, [7]shall we?" Carlos elided with a smile. Of course, he had stopped walking before he posited this question.

"Awesome idea. Thank you so much, I really need to get those photos taken and this will save me a butt load of money on investigating possibilities." With that, I listened to Carlos introduce idea after idea

---

7   Bresciani, M.J. (2011). *Rushing to Yoga.* Bloomington, IN:Balboa Press.

for the cover of the book. We strolled from one gorgeous Coronado location to another, using his I–Phone for practice photos. I had a blast. *I wonder if Jesus was this fun.*

After completing the sample photos and ruling out several ideas, I offered to buy Carlos a cup of tea in gratitude for the generous sharing of his creativity. *I wonder if Jesus was creative.* Carlos warmly accepted and of course insisted that we first return to my Jeep so he could use his own tea mug. *I wonder if Jesus was green.*

After ordering the tea, I asked Carlos if he would mind if we drank it on the run. After all, this request would mean I would be asking him to do two things at once. I explained to him that in the midst of enjoying my time with him, I had lost track of time and was now late for meeting Katerina for yoga class. He graciously agreed. I asked him random questions on the way back to the seminar and he left me with wise short questions in response. I was smiling the entire drive back to the seminar location.

After dropping off Carlos at his car, I called Katerina to explain why I was running late. "I am sorry Katerina, I know I am late. And I am sorry that I didn't even let you know I was going to be late. I was so distracted. I had Jesus in my Jeep."

Gracious Katerina let out a delicate howl, let me know that the later yoga class was actually more convenient for her as she had been running late caused by something that clearly was not going to be as amusing as what I had experienced. And we chatted a little while longer.

As I hung up the phone and made my way to pick up Katerina, I looked over to my now empty passenger seat. It was still radiating with love from its prior occupant. *Was that really what it was like to hang out with Jesus or Buddha or Gandhi or any of the great Masters in living and teaching Love? Or was that just what it was like to hang out with a person who was committed to choosing love in every moment that he could?*

I didn't know but I sent out the intention and therefore the invitation to the Universe to remain open to learning lessons that maybe, for me, had to be learned in pain. And I sent out gratitude along with the invitation to the Universe that I would like to spend more time in the

Jesus was in My Jeep

company of her Masters or at the very least in the company of those who chose love moment-by-moment. And then I realized that I had just sent out an invitation to the Universe inviting me, along with each one of us to enjoy the company of each other as if we are mutually and simultaneously both Master and student.

CHAPTER THREE

Exploring the Holy Relationship

Hey Thomas,

I hope you are getting some rest today. I look forward to hearing more about your perspective on the conversations we had about what a holy relationship is and what about the conversation exhausted you. I trust it is one of those "good" exhaustions.

I am sorry I had to cut you off quickly on the phone. I am not skilled at staying present on a phone call while I board a plane. :)

I wanted to explain why I invited my sister along on our hike. Actually, I haven't invited her yet; I wanted to make sure it was OK with you first. I wanted to invite my sister along on our hike for three reasons. 1) I think the exposure to the types of conversation we will have will open more doors for her to explore as she begins and continues her own spiritual journey. You don't have to censor anything you want to say around her and I won't either. Cool beans? 2) I wanted her to see what a handsome, successful man who is open to exploring spirituality looks like. I wanted her to see that "good" men exist and that they can have spiritual conversations and still be "all man". And 3) after much reflection about the holy relationship, the honoring of the God in others and within ourselves, and the resonating out of thoughts, words, and actions, I need to <u>not </u>spend alone time with you. What I mean is that it wasn't resonating well with me to spend alone time with you hiking (a very spiritual connecting activity for me) and *talking about spiritual stuff (another intimate activity). I mean, if I were cool with us just being friends - no worries. After all, that is what I did with Kaila all weekend (hiking in the Redwoods and bunches of spiritual conversations) but I am not attracted to her. I mean I love her very much and would do anything for her but I am not the least bit attracted to her. Knowing that I am attracted to you and knowing that you are in a committed relationship, I feel that I can best show up in a friendship to you when other people are around. That way, our time together will be shared with others and we can all enjoy each other's beauty and lessons. And I won't be tempted to physically connect with you as I would if I were alone with you.*

So, the bottom line for me Thomas is that I look forward to more conversations with you. And in order for me to feel that I am showing up in truth and honor, I need for us to have those conversations in the presence of others. Does that make sense?

My best, Marilee

"So, yeah, that is the email that I sent to him. What do you think?" I excitedly asked my dear friend Ivina after I could tell from the look in her eyes that she had finished reading it. I was anxiously awaiting to hear what I expected would be an encouraging reply.

She stared a little while longer at the email displayed proudly on my laptop, looked up at me, looked back down at the email, glanced back up at me, and then she reached for her glass of lemonade that was resting on my kitchen counter next to my overworked laptop. Ivina's hesitation to reply gave me an opportunity to sit back in my bar stool and prepare for what I now expected would no longer be an encouraging response.

"I think you are lying." She said softly in between sips of her lemonade.

"I am what?" I lurched forward in my bar stool so quickly that I almost thrust myself right out of it.

"Come on Marilee, that email is bullshit. If you really wanted to honor the woman he is dating, you wouldn't even have agreed to another hike with him. You know he also has an interest in you. Your last hike revealed plenty of evidence of that. This is not about honoring anyone. This is about you feeling like you are coming clean while fully investing in your desire to spend more time with him in a chaperoned environment."

Ivina shared all of this without much emotion and without even setting down her glass of lemonade. I didn't feel judged. I just felt like she was calling it like she saw it. *She is so amazing.*

"Iveenahhhh" I moaned like a 2-year old trying to get some sympathy after just having fallen with a scraped knee. "How am I suppose to learn about what a holy relationship looks like if I no longer can have a conversation with an intelligent man to whom I am attracted and who also is exploring this concept?"

Ivina glanced over at me with a look that reflected something more resonant of a question – similar to just asking her a question like, "how on earth did I get a scraped knee after falling down three flights of concrete stairs?" I got the picture. She didn't need to say anything more.

Ivina was right. I knew she was right, but now, I didn't know what to do about her being right. I was just filled with questions. After some additional light conversation, Ivina left. I returned to my journal to write. My pen wrote out random questions and then attempted to answer them.

1) What need or desire does an exclusive dating relationship satisfy? Perhaps none; perhaps it just represents an honoring of a commitment. Or perhaps it satisfies a need for security. I have no idea.

2) Can a desire to be held or to hold someone be unholy if no expectations exist beyond the embrace? However, what if desires arises when you are holding someone? Is the embrace now made unholy? I have no idea.

3) How do you "wait and see" what will happen in a relationship if you have no desires or intentions? Isn't that an oxymoron in and of itself? Isn't "wait and see" only for those who really do have expectations and they are waiting to see if their expectations are realized? OK, this one, this one seems to make more sense. So I must really not know what I am talking about here.

4) If we focus on constantly being in the moment, where does commitment come into play? Can we be fully committed to another in a partnership and be fully in the moment all the time? Yes, I think that makes sense. Therefore again, I must really not know what I am talking about.

5) Rather than a suppression of desire, would a holy relationship be about a union where desires and wants are felt and communicated. However, the desires and wants are not expected to be met by the other? OK, that also makes sense, but then I think that would be called the impossible relationship, rather than the Holy relationship. That was funny.

Yet, I think, in this moment, this is what I understand a holy relationship to be. I think it is communicating to each other wants and needs and then understanding when the other is unable or unwilling to meet those wants and needs. In that moment when the other is unable or unwilling to meet my wants and needs, rather than projecting onto the other person resentment and blame, I tend to my own wants and needs without judgment of the other and without resentment. In the end, I don't think this is nearly as difficult to comprehend as I have been making it out to be.

I have a desire, but I don't have an expectation. I don't have peace around that because I am aware of this unfulfilled desire. I thought I would feel better about it if I spoke it, but it seems to have only fueled it. Damn. I trust that in time, the desire will dissolve or I will surrender to the desire or I will choose to let it go. And until then (dissolution, surrender, or letting go), I will make sure that chaperones are around when I spend time with Thomas. Everyone deserves honor and respect for we are all connected and we are all children of God. What I choose affects others. Even though I am responsible for tending to my own needs and desires, if I do so without being cognizant of how my choices affect others in my life, I am not showing up in love. And therefore, I am not recognizing that the Holy Spirit reside in others and thus, I am not engaged in holy relating. I choose the Holy Relationship for all of my relationships.

CHAPTER FOUR

I am In-Authentic

"I am what?" I declared aloud with the microphone in hand, standing in front of 160 people, only 8 of them I had actually remembered the names of from our one-hour "meet and greet" the night prior.

"You are inauthentic. You are what I call 'a concern for looking good.'" The yoga master's voice boomed over his headset microphone, filling the auditorium where I, along with 160 other people, had just completed a morning meditation and were preparing for a 4 hour yoga practice at our week-long yoga teacher training located on the Big Island of Hawaii.

I was pissed and I was shaking. I did not just spend over $3,000 and a week of vacation during a very busy time of year to be insulted in public in front of over 160 people I didn't even know. *Why had I signed up for this yoga retreat anyway? What an asshole this guy was. He has no idea of what I have just been through or who I am. Who is he to call me inauthentic? I think he is projecting his own in-authenticity. I am going to give him a lecture he will never forget.*

Wait a minute; if I am even thinking like this, he just may have something here. Maybe I should remove my hand from my cocked hip and listen a little bit longer. OK, that seems like a good idea. After all, you paid over 3k for this, make the asshole work for his money.

Even though I thought I was preparing to learn from this yoga master, the ass-hole inside of me arose and spoke up, "I am WHAT?" Yes, I am pretty sure I yelled back at him even though I didn't really intend to do so. And then I noticed that my hand was still on my cocked hip with the other hand holding the microphone. *Oopsie.*

"You are inauthentic; you are a concern for looking good. You care more about how your message will be received than you care about delivering the message that you have actually been given to deliver." Baron Baptiste [8] responded calmly and seemingly disinterested in the pain that I was now experiencing from hearing his words.

"OUCH!" I exclaimed aloud into the mic I was apparently still holding up to my mouth and as I did so, the tears began to make their way out of my eyeballs and onto my cheeks. *Stop that; don't let this guy see you cry. He will have won then. Pull it together; don't let him mind fuck you. Be strong; say something funny or smart.*

"If I am so inauthentic, why am I crying right now?"

Oh my god, is that the best you can do? That was neither funny nor smart. Holy shit! You are looking like a total idiot in front of all these people. My mind was yelling at my body to pull it together but my body wasn't listening. I began to shake and the tears were streaming down my face uncontrollably. *Inauthentic? How could I be inauthentic when everyone in my life was telling me to quit living so out loud, so public. How could I be inauthentic when I had just lost friends I adore because they didn't like this new way in which I was showing up?*

It was as if he read my mind.

"I don't care about the changes you have already made in your life. I don't care that you think you have arrived. You haven't. You are successful, yet you are here. Why are you here?"

Fucking damn good question. But at least this time, I didn't say it aloud into the microphone. I was still shaking and still crying. The manic rage of self-judgment and defensiveness was building inside me. *Why am I here? This is insane. I don't need to be treated like this. Why am I here?*

---

8   Baron Baptiste, Founder of Baron Baptiste Power Vinyasa Yoga Institute - http://baronbaptiste.com/

His words kept interrupting the chatter in my head.

"You are a success. Of course you are. Everything you have done thus far in your life has gotten you everything you have and everything you have not." Baron spoke these words to me calmly and peacefully. I could tell he was trying to coach me back into authenticity in a firm and loving manner; a manner I was not used to experiencing.

Huh? OK, now you have my attention. Yes, that is why I am here. I am successful. I am happy, yet I am still aware of what I do not have, which is peace and I have no fucking clue how to get it. I am on the hamster wheel knowing full well that in order to be perceived as successful, I have to produce and produce and produce. I love what I do but I am not at peace. I feel driven and I am running. I am tired and I can't rest. I am here to get help.

"And you are still a concern for looking good, so what can you let go of?"

What can I let go of?

"I can let go of this fucking microphone." I announced proudly into the mic that I so desperately wanted to drop to the ground.

OK, that was funny! But why was no one laughing? Come on everyone, I pleaded with my eyes, as I looked out onto the mass of people, no longer able to distinguish individual faces as the tears were blocking all vision. *That was funny. Why is no one laughing? Holy shit, is that what he means by my still being a concern for looking good?*

I turned back to Baron and pleaded into the shaking microphone that I was very aware of still holding. "I would really rather you all be laughing at me right now. Instead I am up here crying. Furthermore, I don't even understand your question."

He asked it again. "What can you let go of?"

My face contorted into several painful shapes. I had no idea what he was asking and therefore I had no idea of the answer. I wasn't feeling smart or funny, apart from fighting the need to ask him if he was aware that he kept ending sentences with prepositions.

No, I wasn't feeling funny. I was feeling naked. I focused my attention on the hand that was not clutching the mic and realized that it was no longer on my hip. It was dangling helplessly by my side;

helplessness was the feeling that was resonating throughout my entire body. I was feeling so helpless and naked that I asked my hand to touch my legs to see if I actually was wearing clothes. I was; the realization of which gave me new courage.

"I don't understand what you are asking." I sheepishly and honestly replied.

He quickly bent over, grabbed a yoga block from the floor, and stood back up. He extended his arm holding the yoga block and then he simply dropped it.

"What can you let go of?" He announced again. "Just as I let go of this block, what can you let go of?"

My mind began to play with retorts that I was sure would make the crowd laugh. I was playing around in my head with responses like; *did you know you keep ending sentences with prepositions?* And *Letting go of a yoga block is a hell of a lot easier than letting go of 46 years of programming. Besides, thank you so much for not throwing that block at me, which is what I thought you were going to do when you bent over to pick it up. Where the hell did that thought come from? I think I am losing my mind right here in front of everyone.*

Holy spirit, please help me.

Finally I prayed the prayer that made a difference and out of my mouth came an answer.

"I don't know of what I can let go. Can you please give me a clue?" *That was not very smart, even though you modeled not ending the sentence with a preposition.* My evil twin told my shaking body. *You are so going to get humiliated for that question.* Yet, in spite of my mind chatter, I realized that in asking that question as a response to prayer, my eyes stopped weeping and my body stopped shaking.

"Thank you for asking" he replied.

Oh my god, did he just thank me?

"You can let go of the need to know. You can let go of trying to fix yourself. You can let go of trying to find the answer." He said it all so confidently, so assuredly, so peacefully.

But what did I do? My mind screamed again in response to his thoughtful questions. *Let go of what? Let go of my brain? I don't think so. Is this a cult? What is going on here anyway? Let go of what?*

Fortunately, my mind didn't speak. I was still in prayer asking the Holy Spirit to help me see this differently.

"I don't know how to do that." I replied honestly and authentically, and with a feeling of complete terror of this new unknown.

"Well, don't try to figure out how." He responded with a loving smirk. (Yes, loving smirks do exist in the world and they are really quite charming when you encounter them.) With that, I got to let go of the mic and take my seat. Niagara falls returned to my eyes as I plopped down like Jell-O onto my yoga mat at the northwest corner of the large auditorium.

I don't know how to let go. He just gave me the answer *and I don't know how to implement it. On top of that, I just humiliated myself in front of 160 people with whom I have to spend 6 more days. I wonder if I can crawl under this yoga mat, hide for 6 days where no one can see me. Or better yet, maybe I can quit and go take a much-needed vacation. I won't even care if they never refund my money.*

"Let's take a ten minute break and come back onto your mats into downward dog." I heard his assistant announce.

What? We are breaking? Now? I am so fucked. I don't even have time to sneak out of here and hide. Through the drying of my tears on my yoga towel, I saw my small group teammates (5 of the 8 names I knew) beeline their way toward me with arms opened wide for loving embraces. There will be no quitting today; no possibility of hiding; only a challenge from 160 people to make sure I show up in authenticity and learn how to let go. *I have a feeling that I am going to more than get my money's worth out of this week.*

As my team members embraced me one-by-one in acknowledgement of my courage to stand and share. Snuggled into their loving embrace of my now obvious pain, I cried even more. *How could they be this generous and this open with their love? They just met me briefly last night. We spent like 45 minutes together.* My mind continued to cling to words that echoed as if they had been shouted in the Grand Canyon. *There will be no more hiding. You have been identified as inauthentic. What can you now let go of?* Or perhaps, as my ego kept screaming still trying to have its voice heard, *of what can you now let go?*

CHAPTER FIVE

Before Surrender, Acceptance

"What comes first?" Baron Baptiste's voice boomed into the microphone, which was actually an amazing feat because I had earlier been thinking that the sound system sort of sucked. Then again, maybe it wasn't the sound system; maybe it was my way of listening that was short of being excellent.

Yup, I wasn't listening. I didn't even know what he was asking. *What comes first in what? In the yoga sequence? In what? Uh-oh... I don't know what the question means. I don't even know what he asked?* And since we had promised not to cross-talk during the lecture time, I couldn't even lean over to my colleague to ask her for help. So, I glanced down at her journal. *Damn,* she hadn't written the question down.

"What comes first in your steps to begin feeling the way you want to feel?" he repeated.

Thank god he reads minds. And yeah, I guess the sound system is fine; I can now hear him perfectly. It was I. Go figure.

He continued, "What comes first in determining who you need to be in order to feel the way you want to feel, versus determining what you need to do in order to feel the way you need to feel?"

Well, I had never thought of that before. And so now that I knew what his question was, I didn't feel any better. I still didn't know what the question meant. Not really anyway. *What does he mean?*

Hands shot up from all my fellow yogis. They were each taking their turns speaking their answers into the microphone and each time he would respond, "Good answer, but no." Sometimes he would even question them further to get at what they were really trying to say before he would tell them no.

I know, I know. My mind convinced my arm, so my arm shot up in the air with greater energy than I realized I even possessed at this point in the yoga boot camp.

But then someone else spoke my answer. "Letting go of judgment of self."

"Good answer, but no." Baron responded.

With that reply, my arm fell to my side with such gravitational defeat that it almost hit me in the head on its way down back to my side… as if to say, *stupido, why did you think you knew the answer when you still don't even understand the question?*

One after one, people would raise their hands. Hands continued to shoot up and down with rapid pace with each yogi's reply. *There are 160 of us. If everyone wants to have a shot at this, this is going to take some time.* I began to settle back into my chair preparing for some rest as I had already given up on knowing what the answer was. I kept comforting myself with my confusion, making excuses about how I wasn't sure that I even understood the question.

In the moment that I had just gotten comfortable in my chair, he spoke again.

"Incorrect answer after answer yogis and you still seek the answer. Why is that?"

Yes, now this question I understood and I could answer this one. So I shot my hand back up in the air. But he chose some else and they spoke my answer.

"Our ego wants to be right." One of my priceless yogi colleagues announced loudly and confidently into the microphone. She beamed, but he just stared blankly at her.

What? No "good answer" response? That was a good answer. Why isn't he telling her that that was a good answer? It was as if he read my mind again.

He smiled softly as he replied to all of us. "None of you yogis like not knowing, do you?"

My mind was screaming inside. *What? I know. I know tons of stuff. You just don't ask very clear questions. That was a good answer. Why wasn't that a good answer?*

"That is a challenge for you yogis, isn't it? You don't like not knowing."

Baron was peacefully smiling at the front of the room. My heart and head were pounding. *I really hate not knowing. I mean I really, really hate not knowing.*

Baron continued, "The next step in your being what you want to feel is not "doing" what will get you to the way you want to feel. It is in accepting the barrier that keeps you from being the feeling that you desire."

Huh? Am I not listening again or did that just go way over my head? I think that went way over my head. I have no idea what he is saying again.

"So, get out your journals yogis and write this down, 'what is keeping you from being your desired feeling?'"

I grabbed my pen and wrote the question down quickly in my journal. It was at least, something I could do. As I stared down at the question, my mind continued its frantic chatter.

OK, so I want to feel peace, what is keeping me from feeling peace? I get it I get it. It is my need to know. My need to figure out every blessed thing is keeping me from being peace. Got it! Yay me, yay me. Now, what do I do?

"Once you have written down the barrier that is keeping you from being that which you want to feel, embrace it, accept it, be with it, 100%."

What? I have to accept being in a place of not knowing? No fucking way.

"I want each of you to partner up and make a commitment to your yogi partner that you will accept your barrier, whatever it is 100%. I want you to state that you are for this state of being 100% as it is or as it is not."

What? I have to be for a state of not knowing 100%? I can't do this. I can't accept being in a place of not knowing. I don't want to be in a place of not knowing. Who would want to be OK about being in a place of not knowing? This is insane.

As I partnered with my colleague and we shared our barriers, my colleague assured me that if I didn't believe what I was saying, then I really didn't accept my barrier and if I didn't really accept my barrier, then I was not on my way to letting it go. That pissed me off even more. I knew he was right. And I didn't know what to do about it. So, I told him I needed a moment by myself so that my *will* could have a conversation with my *mind*.

Will: *OK, mind. I have the intention to be peaceful and loving so get out of my way and quit trying to figure out everything all the time. Quit trying to manage everything around you so that you come off looking good. Just get out of my way so I can be at peace. OK?*

Mind: *Nope*

Will: *What? What do you mean "nope"? I really want to be at peace and be loving so quit trying to figure out everything and just rest in knowing you don't know anything and aren't going to be able to figure it out at all. OK?*

Mind: *Nope*

Will: *OK mind, you are really pissing me off here. I can't get past day two assignments at this yoga boot camp if you don't start cooperating. I need you to cooperate. I explained to you what I need you to do and why I need for you to cooperate so will you cooperate now?*

Mind: *Nope.*

Will: *What? Why not? Can't you see the pain you are causing me and the body in which you reside?*

Mind: *Yup*

Will: *Then why won't you cooperate and let go of your need to know? It will advance my ability to be peace, joy, and love?*

Mind: *It is a lot of fun fucking with all ya'll.*

Will: *What? We are supposed to be connected. We are supposed to be one – mind, body, and soul. So come on, be a good team player. Will you please?*

Mind: *Listen missy good intentions, you have spent the majority of your life feeding your intellect. You love being in the know; you love how powerful it makes you feel to know something or to be able to figure it out and to know where to go to find out an answer when you don't know the answer. You have spent your life creating me to be like this. So, now, you are experiencing some sort of retreat and trying to get to a place of peace and just because you desire this, you expect me to just shut up, turn off, and allow it to happen? You are crazy. I ain't going to let you shut me down after you have spent most of your life creating me to manage everything in your life.*

Will: *You think pretty highly of yourself, don't you?*

Mind: *You should know that is true, that is what you intended when you spent so much time focusing on my development. I have become what you made me to become, why would you be angry with me now that you want me to shut down?*

Will: *I don't want you to shut down mind; I just want to challenge you in a new way. I want you to practice being OK with not knowing. I want to stretch you in a way I never have before by asking you to sit in a place of not knowing for just one moment. Just to try on something new, to see how it feels to sit in a place of not knowing before you try to figure out what to do or what to say or search for more answers. Consider it a new test of your capacity.*

Mind: *What capacity? It takes no capacity of mine to be in a place of not knowing.*

Will: *Well, if it takes no capacity, why are you resisting?*

Mind: *I don't want to rust from lack of use.*

Will: *You're insane.*

Mind: *All minds are insane; some of us just hide it better than others.*

Will: *I dare you to try it. I dare you to investigate what it feels like to not know for just an instant. Who knows? Maybe some new cranial space will open up from your attempting to try something you never have before…like being honest in admitting you don't know something and then just sitting with it for a while. What do you think? Will you try it for just an instant?*

Mind: *For just an instant? I can <u>do</u> that easily. Here we go.*

Marilee: *Hey, I am in not knowing again. Cool. Can I accept just for this moment that I don't even know how to accept being in a state of not knowing? Can I be OK for it for just this moment? Well, for this moment, I can. Oops, now I am not OK. OK, now I am OK with it again. Oopsie, now I am not.*

I realized that this was going to take some practice and some conscience moment-by-moment choices. I also was acutely aware that if I didn't try being something different than what I had come to know, than I would never realize all that I can be and become. So, I began again turning my conscience to my choices.

OK, now I am OK with not knowing again. Oopsie, now I am not. Oh, I am OK again. Ugh, now I am not... Yup, this is going to be a moment-to-moment journey.

CHAPTER SIX

Letting Go

"I have no fucking clue how to let go of anything except an electric fence and … oh yeah, a barbed wire fence. THAT," I exclaimed aloud to my priceless friend and colleague, Leanna, "I know how to do."

She laughed heartily, her full body shaking. Her lightness to my sincere response made me smile. I needed that.

Leanna laughed again as she read over my workshop evaluations. "Well that might explain why participant after participant commented about how you need to expand more on explaining the concept of 'letting go' in your workshops. They say they don't fully understand it."

I looked over at Leanna as she was pouring over approximately 200 evaluations with great care. Leanna was so good at helping me distill evaluations down into succinct "to do" lists of what I specifically needed to focus on next in order to improve my workshops. I so appreciated her many gifts.

Sighing as if my breath was carrying the weight of the world, I responded to Leanna's comment.

"Well, that makes sense, doesn't it Lee? I mean, I keep telling folks that I am sharing what I need to learn. So, if I haven't learned it, I can't share it clearly. Can I?" Another heavy sigh accompanied with a grunt came flooding out of my body as my bum hit the office chair almost as heavy as my breath.

"Frick!" I yelled out startling Leanna so much that she tossed a pile of evaluations that she had been going through in the air. "These hotel office chairs are getting harder and harder. I gotta be more careful with how I sit down in them." With that comment, we burst into laughter. It was a welcomed diversion from my prior string of self-judgments.

Leanna scrambled to gather the evaluations she had just flung into mid air while I opened my laptop to review my workshop outline. I wanted to 'fix" the workshop right away. I wanted to make it all better immediately. As I began to pour over the intricate design of the workshop looking to tweak every detail, my mind began its own conversation with itself. For some people, this may sound odd. For me, my mind chats occur every day and sometimes several times a day.

What are you doing?

I am trying to fix this workshop so that I can show folks how to "let go".

Uh-huh. Right. Any insanity coming to you in all of that "doing"?

Huh? What? I don't get it.

Hello? Any insanity coming to you? You are trying to "do" something to "fix" something that requires no "doing" or "fixing". Am I making any sense now?

Uh...uh...uh...

I said, you are trying to "fix" something in a "doing" workshop to illustrate to people how to "let go". You don't see any irony in that?

"I am an idiot," I exclaimed aloud, yet thinking that I was still in my little mind conversation.

I startled Leanna with my exclamation once again but this time no papers flew into the air. "What?" she patiently questioned.

"Nothing" I said rather embarrassed that the thoughts in my mind had actually come out of my mouth. *I hate it when that happens.* "I am sorry to have disturbed you again." I apologized sincerely to Leanna and then returned to my thoughts but this time, my mind was quieter.

Letting go; yes, letting go requires no doing. Not really. It only requires, acknowledgement, genuine acceptance and then moment-by-moment release.

This type of letting go is a whole different notion of doing than I am accustomed to understanding. I am accustomed to the kind of doing that incorporates "work your ass off all hours of the day" kind of doing. I am accustomed to the "you want it? Then, roll up your sleeves and work for it" kind of doing. Don't know the answer? Go find it. Don't like how the person around you is acting, then manipulate or manage him into a place where you are more likely to tolerate him.

Letting go? That is more of a well, just that. Acknowledge what you want to let go, honestly accept what you want to let go of as it is or is not 100%, and then release it sincerely and genuinely moment by moment.

That's it. That's the part I keep forgetting. It is a moment-by-moment decision to let go. It is not some one-time act or even daily act. It is a moment-by-moment decision. *Holy Moses, no wonder this is so elusive for me.* It doesn't require a regimen or a plan, it requires me to be awake, to be conscious of what is going on within me and around me and to release it in a single moment – one moment at a time. *Ha! I guess we are back to that whole staying in the moment thing again. Funny how it always comes back to that, isn't it? Funny indeed.*

CHAPTER SEVEN

Releasing an Un-Holy Relationship

"Thank you Elisa. You are such an angel. Thank you for asking. Well, I don't know. I don't know how it is going with Thomas and me." I realized as I responded to Elisa's question that my shoulders lost their energy and I had slumped forward in my chair. I was now feeling energetically disempowered as I sat across the table from her.

"Hey, you OK?" she perked up in her chair as if to hold the space with enough energy for both of us. It worked. In her response, I found energy to sit taller and pull my shoulders back, regaining my own personal seated Tadasana position[9].

"Thank you gorgeous. Thank you. Honestly, I don't know what 'OK' means so how about I just share how I feel?" I smiled. As I responded, I began to energetically straighten my spine, and physically adjust my shoulder blades back and down in order to feel more fully in Tadasana. I then took three slow, full breaths. As a result, I felt that I

---

9 Tadasana – a yoga asana or position that involves standing at attention. To get into that asana, stand firmly on both feet with all corners of your feet firmly planted on the earth. Tuck your buttocks and expand upward from your spine. Square your chest with your shoulders rolled back and relaxed. Imagine that your neck is an extension of your spine as energy radiates upward from the foundation of your feet through the top of your head. This is a "stand in your authenticity, knowing the source of your power" kind of pose.

had stepped fully back into my power even though I remained seated. It felt good.

"Of course you dork. That is what I was asking. Tell me how your heart feels." She smiled back as she spoke. Her playful taunting made me feel lighter.

"Thanks Elisa. Great question. Well, here it goes."

I re-capped for myself much more than for Elisa, for she had already known that Thomas had chosen to no longer date the woman he was dating when we met. We then decided that since we were mutually attracted to each other and since he decided to no longer date the woman he was dating when we met, we might as well start dating each other. A no-brainer decision as my friends would call it.

My friends adored Thomas and so did I. He was funny, confident, very bright, handsome, fun, wise, and I could have the much-desired spiritual conversations that I really wanted to have with a man, especially one with whom I was falling in love. Yet, something was not resonating well within me. I kept feeling like I was the one who was always learning; like I was the one who had so much that needed to be improved upon in the relationship. I thought that perhaps it was because I needed to learn lessons that only he could teach me.

What I mean by that is that I had made a recent commitment to come out of my comfort zone and move into a place of not knowing. In that place, I wanted to discover the lessons that could be learned as I faced my blind spots, as I faced a state of not knowing and a state of not needing to know. However, recently, my discomfort was growing.

"Thomas has recently immersed himself in studying the Tao."

"Cool," Elisa piped in.

"Yeah," I responded with far less enthusiasm than Elisa had shared. I continued. "Last night we had a brief phone conversation; by brief, I mean very brief. He shared one of the verses in the Tao to me, which basically had to do with letting things go and letting relationships flow as they will. I told him I was not feeling well, which I wasn't. I mean I can't believe my sinus infection is back so soon. So, I didn't want to talk anymore about anything. My throat was almost swollen shut after a night of teaching. So, this morning I studied the verse he quoted to me last night in Wayne Dyer's [10]book entitled "Change your Thoughts, Change your Life."

"Cool," Elisa shouted again. "Did he share this verse with you in response to your query to him about why he had withdrawn and what he was thinking so much about?"

"Yeah, I think that was his teaching point." I remarked with a bit of sarcasm. "Well, Wayne's words landed on me better than Thomas's did. Perhaps because I am not regularly making out with Wayne Dyer." I burst into laughter at what I thought was my obvious keen sense of humor, however Elisa didn't laugh. So, when my solo laughter died down, I continued.

"In any event, here is where we are. The thoughts that have been occupying Thomas this past week are thoughts that he does not want to share with me. And he thinks I shouldn't make up stories for why he does not want to share them. I think he makes a good point there, as that is exactly what I was doing. I was thinking that I am not as 'evolved' spiritually as he is and he is probably just tired of having to teach me all the time. I made up other stories too but that is the best one so far. In any event, he told me that he likes to teach me and he likes to teach others, but he doesn't want to share the thoughts he turns around and around in his head with me. My choice is that I can continue to ask him why he doesn't share his thoughts with me and he will continue to not answer. Or I can let it go. I choose to let that line of questioning go."

"Well, how does that feel?" Elisa wisely questioned, forking into her mouth another taste of her favorite four-cheese lobster macaroni and cheese delicacies from one of our favorite San Diego hangouts.

"I don't know how I feel about being in relationship with someone who asks me about my thoughts yet doesn't share his. Honestly, my first thought is that it sucks; that it feels off-balance but my second thought is this is great. If I feel so uncomfortable about this, I must have something to learn from this. Yet, I don't know. I just don't know. What the fuck

10 Dyer, W. (2007). *Change Your Thoughts - Change Your Life: Living the Wisdom of the Tao.* Carlsbad, CA:Hay House Inc.

33

is it that I am suppose to be learning?" My voice became a little loud with emotion as I spoke. Elisa paused just a moment and then piped in before I could start again.

"Honestly Marilee, do you always have to use the 'f' word and use it so loudly?"

"*That* question? *That* question I know the answer to and the answer is YES!" I yelled out so loudly that now Elisa was hunched over in her chair as if trying to hide from the many folks who were now looking our way.

I thought I was funny again, and I didn't care who was looking our way or why. I had enough on my mind. Yet, I knew I had gotten a little loud from being caught up in my own personal drama so I lowered my voice and continued.

"My April 4th Conversations with God [11]daily reading said, 'you have no obligation in relationship. You have only opportunity. Opportunity, not obligation is the cornerstone of religion, the basis of spirituality. So long as you see it the other way around, you will have missed the point.'

Elisa's face contorted trying to understand what I was saying. I was trying to understand what I was saying so her face contortion was so not helpful. But I took it as encouragement that I was not the only one confused by my thoughts; that thought was very helpful and very comforting.

"Elisa, I think Thomas is my opportunity to practice letting go of relationship obligations. In this moment right now, to me that also means letting go of relationship commitments. But maybe obligation and commitment do not go hand in glove. Maybe commitment and opportunity go hand in glove. I have no idea. For now, all I know is I am practicing letting go of relationship obligations. I guess I will see what happens to commitment along the way. What a fascinating learning opportunity. Huh?" I was trying my best to be excited about this newfound learning opportunity.

---

11   Walsch, N.D. (1997) *Meditations from Conversations with God.* Charlottesville, VA: Hampton Roads Publishing.

Elisa was not convinced. She wisely responded with a question.

My friends and I had committed to communicating in inquiry. This was not always easy to do because we often found ourselves having to stop our judgmental words in order to reframe things to inquiry. Our intention was to open ourselves to possibilities we had never yet experienced before. It really was fun, even though it was taking us longer and longer to communicate.

"And how does that make you feel?" she responded.

I paused and then I began to giggle. I was thinking about the doctor's appointment that I had earlier that day. I knew I had a sinus infection (ironically, it was the second sinus infection I had had after meeting Thomas) and I didn't want to go to the doctor but I had to get on a plane soon, which meant I had to get some drugs to get the infection down so the pain would be more manageable in flight. Elisa looked up from her lobster mac and cheese with a worried expression at the delay of my response. Watching her gooey pasta fall from her fork onto her plate made me giggle louder and I blurted out. "Icky oozy."

"Icky oozy?" Elisa questioned, now even more concerned about my emotional state.

"Yeah," I giggled as I re-told the story of the doctor's visit that day and the expression the doctor had made when she peered into my nasal cavity. We both laughed at the thought of a highly trained medical doctor making that kind of comment as she peered into someone's nose. It really was hilarious and it was rather telling of my emotional state as well. Coincidence? I think not.

"So, yeah Elisa, it doesn't feel good." We sat in silence for a while. I was grateful that she asked me how I felt. It allowed me a moment to get out of my head about how I thought I was suppose to feel about a learning opportunity and the practice of letting go. Her question put me back in touch with how I really felt about the practice of letting go. After a very long while, I spoke again.

"I guess I am sad. I don't want to let go. I want to answer my calling to step into my authenticity but this... this lesson feels icky." We sat in silence a little longer. I broke the silence with more of my thoughts.

"Elisa, I am not clear about how many of these teachings we have been studying connect. I understand the process of inviting in my desires so that I can manifest my dreams and co-create my reality. I understand the process of allowing, and getting to a place of higher resonance with what is happening in my life. I understand the practice of re-framing by focusing on the difference between fact and interpretation. I understand about the process of letting go. I don't understand how they all connect. I mean, I desire a husband, I desire kids, and I desire grandchildren. Yet, more than anything I desire being of the spirit world and being connected to God/the Universe/the Higher Power/whatever folks want to call it. I desire being love, being of love, and loving others completely. And in my being, I desire to bring others to love as God loves. Does this all only come into my life if I truly let it all go? Or does it come into my life if I set an intention for it? Are my intentions to have a family and be in the service of God in competition? How could love in various forms be in competition? Isn't love just love?"

Elisa's silence echoed mine. Then after a long pause, she looked up at me with an ornery grin.

"What?" I asked expecting her to answer all my questions with one simple word.

She grinned from ear to ear. "I don't know the answers to your questions Marilee. And clearly you don't either. Isn't it great that you are embracing your state of not knowing so fully?"

With that, our laughter echoed throughout the entire beachfront restaurant. We howled so heartily that I had to grab my sides and lay over onto the unoccupied chair beside me. Her response was perfect. When I finally could regain control of my laughing, drying the amused tears from my eyes. I said, "Yeah, time to remember to let the need to know go again. Thank you Elisa. You are a sage."

CHAPTER EIGHT

Not Knowing

"Yes, I really am being serious. There is nothing scary about being in a state of not knowing. Uncomfortable? Hell, yeah. Scary? No, why would it be?" I took another sip of my green tea soy latte, no classic, no foam; my favorite hot Starbucks beverage and then glanced over at my friend Ivina.

Her face was contorted. She had been questioning me about my new state of being – the state of being in "I don't know" – for hours. And I knew I wasn't satisfying her curiosity, but I really had no idea how I was going to be able to do so. Moments, or maybe it had been decades of minutes earlier, I am not really sure, I had explained to her that I was finding it difficult to just be in a place where I wasn't trying to figure out everything, to be in a place where I was accepting not knowing what was coming next.

It was very uncomfortable for me to be there in this state of not knowing. I was so much more comfortable being in a place where I was analyzing the hell out of everything or analyzing the heaven out of it, whatever. I was simply more comfortable trying to figure things out than I was accepting being in a place where I didn't know the answers.

I found myself going back to my beginnings in order to explain to Ivina my inherent need to figure things out for myself. I was explaining to her that I was the kind of kid who would never read directions, never listen to how it should be done regardless of the expert, or even listen to how I could make an activity easier. I had to investigate it all, asking a thousand and one questions on why I needed to read the directions or even do the task. I even had to ask why someone felt that her suggestion would save me time or energy. Yes, my need to know and understand every little detail before doing got me what? Well, as Baron Baptiste [12]would say, it got me to where I am today. That way of being "got me everything I have and everything I have not."

Thus, it brought me to where I was today in my conversation with Ivina, trying on something different. Trying on not knowing for a while in order to discover some of what I have not. So yes, this state was very uncomfortable. Not only was I learning something new by trying not to figure everything out but also I was practicing integrating that into my day-to-day way of being. It felt beyond the discomfort of learning a new habit; it felt more like learning 110 new habits all at the same time.

"What I mean Ivina is that there is nothing scary about being in the state of 'I don't know' because there is an emptiness in that state. It is not an emptiness as in the feeling I have when I feel no hope or the emptiness I feel when in despair; it is more like the emptiness of a creation of space into which something new can flow. Isn't that cool?" I was pretty excited about being in the state of 'I don't know' in that moment, as it did sound pretty adventurous. I so love adventure. However, Ivina looked unconvinced.

"No Marilee, it sounds frightening." Her intensely furrowed brow caused me to chuckle.

"OK, OK, try this on then." I drank the last sip of my green tea soy latte, no classic, no foam, and took the empty cup and held it up to where Ivina could see into it. "What do you see in there Ivina?"

"Remnants of your green tea soy latte. It's gross looking, I can't believe you actually drink something that is green."

---

12   Baron Baptiste, Founder of Baron Baptiste Power Vinyasa Yoga Institute.
     www.baronbaptiste.com

Rolling my eyes, I got up from my seat, walked over to the counter and asked the no doubt over-caffeinated delightfully bright-eyed Starbucks clerk if I could borrow an empty cup. She enthusiastically obliged and assured me that I didn't need to bring it back. Taking the cup in gratitude, I strolled back over to the little table where I had left Ivina sitting.

"OK, Ivina, what do you see in there?" I asked beaming while holding the cup close to her eyes.

"I see a seam." She replied rather proud of herself.

"Thanks smartass. What else do you see?" I remarked in my most earnest of teaching voices.

Ivina smiled and I could tell she had decided to play along. "I see nothing. I see only space in a cup."

"Yes," I cried out startling Ivina and the two elderly women who had just walked by our table. "Yes, that is what I mean. You see only space where something can now enter. That is what the beingness of 'I don't know' feels like. Now, isn't that cool?"

I could tell by the return of Ivina's furrowed brow that she was still not convinced. So, I continued rather excited by the thoughts that were simply coming to me right then and there in that very moment.

"You could fill this cup up with all the 'what if' thoughts that come while being in a state of 'I don't know'. In so doing, that may mean that being in 'I don't know' is scary. I mean, you could say, I don't know what is coming next. What if I am going to lose my job? In so doing, you have filled your I don't know space with a frightening what if. Similarly, you could say, what if my Prince Charming is coming to whisk me away to Italy where I get to write books, garden, drink wine, ride horses, and cook elaborate meals while hosting friends and family in our quaint little villa? Then, I would be filling up the space with an intention."

With the latter remark, Ivina took her index finger and pointed it down her throat. She was making a gagging gesture in her throat. It made me laugh. Ivina couldn't stand it when women talked about needing a man to fulfill their dreams. Recovering from my laughter and seeing the light shine in Ivina's eyes with no sign of the furrowed brow returning, I continued.

"The point is that I could fill up my state of 'not knowing' with 'what if' thoughts of all kinds. Some would bring me fear and some would launch me into plans of action based on a desire to fulfill my intentions. What I am practicing is a state of not knowing. It is uncomfortable for me to practice this because for 46 years prior, I have practiced figuring things out, making plans, and then making them happen or at the very least I have been practicing picking up the pieces after failed plans and planning something new. I have never simply embraced being in 'not knowing.' Is that helpful?"

I could tell Ivina was contemplating what I had just said and I was delighted by her slow and seemingly reluctant head nod. Then she spoke, "so, does this mean your brain checked out?"

Laughing heartily now causing heads to turn in our direction, I responded. "Ivina, I think most people thought my brain checked out decades ago." With that comment, Ivina joined me in my laughter. After we quieted, I continued.

"No, being in a state of not knowing doesn't mean I stop my inquiry, not at all. What I am experiencing is that I ask why and how just as much as I did when I was trying to figure things out. However, in the moment-by-moment choice to let go of needing to figure it out, new space has opened up for new ways of thinking. There is less fear because I simply don't know. There is less anxiety because there is no need to jump on a plan of action. I simply get to stay in a state of inquiry and as such, thoughts I never allowed myself to entertain before enter. The new creative thoughts now enter because before, I was so caught up in trying to find an answer or an action plan, I was so caught up in constantly and frantically managing and manipulating, that there was simply no space for anything new. That part of embracing not knowing is pretty fun actually."

Ivina's brow had furrowed. "I don't get it. If you are having fun, then why are you uncomfortable."

"Damn good question Ivina. I don't know. Perhaps it is because I am refraining from coming to a conclusion, I am refraining from action, I am refraining from planning. All this inquiry with no rendered judgment or action plan is making me uncomfortable." Ivina was laughing again. *I love it when she laughs.*

"So, how do you get any work done if you are being in a place of not knowing?" Ivina retorted with a hint of sarcasm.

"Another good question Ivina. The state of not knowing is not influencing my ability to get house chores completed or papers graded. I am meeting deadlines; all that is no problem. What it seems to be influencing is the openness I have to refining how I lecture, how I am redesigning assignments and workshops and even how I am showing up in my one-on-one meetings with students or broader meetings with my colleagues. I am not sure how to explain it but I feel as if I am more awake, as if I am hearing with a different set of ears, and I am most definitely sharing thoughts and ideas I never entertained prior to this state."

Ivina's silence was welcomed. I was feeling as if I was falling back into a need to explain and figure things out. As such, I felt I was moving farther out of my not knowing state. I took advantage of Ivina's reflective silence by sharing what I was just feeling in that moment. She respectfully agreed to save the rest of her questions for another time. I thanked her for the way she lovingly asked her questions and thanked her for the opportunity for me to share what I was discovering in my experience. And then I ended by telling her a story.

"One of my student's came into see me today. He wanted to let me know that he was growing increasingly frustrated by my 'Hippie' talk. [13]He wanted more concrete structure about what he was supposed to be doing as he wrote his dissertation. The thing is Ivina, when he said

---

13   My student was referring to my coaching him to be more in the present. The
     student was struggling with writing his dissertation. He was not meeting
     the deadlines I had been setting for him – which were similar deadlines I
     was setting for other students' dissertation work. I was coaching him to be
     alert to what he was feeling and thinking and to inquire into from where the
     beliefs that were shaping his inability to write his dissertation were coming.
     He was tired of my coaching him into conscious awareness of his feelings and
     beliefs and then coaching him to change his thoughts to those that were more
     positive and self-empowering.

that, my ego wanted to strike out with explanations of how the 'Hippie' talk had some amazing research behind it. I wanted to explain to him exactly what I was doing and why; why I was pushing him and his peers so hard to inquire, to think in ways they had never yet been exposed to think, and to ultimately take responsibility for the choices they were to make once they had made it through their inquiry processes in writing their dissertations. But I didn't. I surprised myself; I didn't explain it at all. Instead, I asked him what kind of structure he needed from me that was different than the outline, criteria checklist, and rubrics that had [14]already been provided as well as the detailed feedback I had just given him on his third draft. He never answered that question. He left my office after asking for clarification on a couple of the comments I made on his draft. I encouraged him to let me know how better I could support his learning. He said he would let me know. Ivina, I have no idea how I could help him further. I have no idea if my 'Hippie' talk – challenging students into their own self-inquiry processes – will result in heightened inquiry skills for them and their own ability to challenge others into spaces of more creative thinking. Outcomes-based assessment of this process over time will tell, I know, but for now, not knowing makes me uncomfortable."

Ivina didn't look up from her coffee mug. She stared at it in silence for a very long time. In return, I stared at her thinking of how uncomfortable not knowing felt. But at least I knew that it wasn't a scary place to be, not as long as I didn't fill it up with all sorts of scary 'what if' statements and that, at least in this moment, felt good.

---

14   The students I coach in writing their dissertations have detailed outlines and checklists to follow as they write so they can join me in monitoring their personal progress knowing full well what their committee expects of them. Details of this process can be found at http://interwork.sdsu.edu/eddleaders/ community_college/program-requirements/dissertation.html

CHAPTER NINE

Teaching and Learning

"I think I am finally realizing what it means to be both the student and the teacher in life. I mean, I understood what that meant in the context of the classroom; I always learn from my students. However, I don't think I was really getting what that saying meant in life until just now." I interrupted sharing my own thoughts to point excitedly out to the ocean, asking my friend and colleague Sashina to look out as well. I had thought I had seen dolphins, but I hadn't. Perhaps the early morning sunlight or my weary eyes were playing tricks on me. I kept staring out at the spot I thought I had seen them when my friend Sashina spoke.

"Are you trying to re-phrase the already famous saying that when the student is ready, the teacher will emerge?" Sashina replied to my unfinished thought.

"Huh?" I grunted, completely distracted by the ocean and my search to spot the dolphins once again.

"You didn't see any dolphins Marilee. I mean, it's early enough in the morning for them to be spotted but you didn't see any dolphins." Sashina's declarative statement brought my eyes back from the ocean onto her. *She can be so convincing.* Content that she had regained my attention, she continued.

"Are you just saying that when the student is ready, the teacher will emerge?"

"Good one," I chuckled. While I thought she was joking with me, a quick glance back from the ocean, which had recaptured my attention and back to Sashina's expression told me that my words were making less and less sense. So, I started over with an explanation.

I explained to her that what I had experienced in the doctoral classroom every time I walked in was an environment where people expected to learn from each other. We had, after all, intentionally created such a learning opportunity. The students expected to learn from me and from each other and I expected to learn from them. Thus, we had the perfect learning environment; one that was open to inquiry, open to questioning judgment or conclusions and thus one that explored all the possibilities that were created simply by people sharing, through inquiry what they learned and through their challenging others in inquiry about their conclusions.

What I had just recently realized is that that same environment exists in my every day life. I can intentionally create an environment where every experience of every day is an opportunity for me to learn from and also teach whoever crosses my path. While there is no day-to-day life syllabus, planned lecture or engagement activity and while there are no graded activities, or evaluation tools such as rubrics and criteria checklists, there are plenty of opportunities for me to learn my intended spiritual curriculum and practice the skills I desire to embody. I felt it was similar to when one of our students asks a question that is unrelated to what we had planned to teach and we find ourselves spending the rest of class teaching to that question. We don't plan to teach and learn something, but the opportunity presented itself to us. As a result of the presence of opportunity, we teach and learn from what we experienced in that very moment. Life has given me plenty of opportunities to discover that which I didn't even know I needed to learn. Living life is incredible!

After I finished my explanation, Sashimi looked up at me with an ornery smile. "Thank you for that, I hear you, and I think I understand what you are saying. However, how does that fit in with the age old saying that when the student is ready, the teacher will emerge?"

Smiling back, enjoying the invitation to share more, I shared that I thought that, as students, all we needed to do in order for the teacher to emerge was to invite the lesson to be learned into our lives, whether we knew what the lesson we needed to learn was or was not. In addition, we needed to let go of judging who our teacher may be so that we could be open to learning. My teachers have come from many walks of life; they have been many shapes and sizes, of various races, gender, ethnicities, ages, religious backgrounds, educational orientations, and socio-economic status. I have learned great lessons from all of them but only after I let go of judging the form of my teacher. Finally, inviting in our Higher Power, our God, the Holy Spirit, Jesus, whatever our life source is named and asking for wisdom to interpret the lesson as it is intended was also essential for me to learn.

"So, I believe Sashima, that our teacher is always right in front of us in every moment and in every situation. All we have to do is invite in the lesson, refrain from judging the form of the teacher so that we can hear the lesson, and pray[15] for 'right'[16] interpretation of the lesson

---

15   By prayer, I mean setting the intention through request and visioning. So, when I say that "I am praying for thus and so" or "that my pray is whatever it is", I am setting the intention by visioning that which I feel contributes to the greater good. In setting the intention, I am inviting all energy source (yours and those around you, plus all that which is seen and unseen) to join with my energy source (that of God's creation) to manifest that, which is for the greater good. So, I don't want to make my prayer specific for outcomes that only I can see but rather, my prayers are designed around the intention of a larger vision, which incorporates what I do not see. So for example, let's say I pray for a peace-filled environment at my work place. This may mean different things to those whose energy is joining with mine to create it. Thus, I don't have a definition to see peace as I define it, rather I pray for peace as it unfolds in the creation of my energy and intention (prayer) joining with others' energy and intention (answered prayer).

16   By 'right' I mean, that which serves the greater good. The greater good is denoted by that which serves Love; not love in a romantic or individual sense, but love in a connection of all to One sense. In serving the greater good, one individual is not heralded over another or one group over another. The greater good is about advancing the connection of love among all people.

and 'right' wisdom for its application into our lives. Does that make sense?"

Sashima looked out into the ocean for a moment and then back at me. She smiled her ornery smile once again and I knew another fun question would be coming. "Does that mean you are no longer looking for your own personal Buddha to emerge as your special teacher and guide?"

Laughing heartily at Sashima's question, I had to let her know that it was a great question. She was so right in asking it for months earlier, I had been obsessed with finding the form that would emerge as my next teacher; the teacher who would lead me into surrendering to my call. It took me a while before I could stop laughing long enough to affirm to her that indeed this realization would keep me from looking for my own personal Buddha. Now, I saw Buddha, Jesus, and God in everyone I met; in everyone I saw. They were all my teachers and I was their student. Likewise, I could "pray" for wisdom to discern whether I had a role in sharing anything with them and in so doing, be like a teacher to them. And the cool thing is that all this classroom learning was free, no need to pay tuition, no need to take out loans, it happened in every moment of every day if I was open enough and willing to learn.

Sashima smiled one last time at my last shared comment about all this learning being free and she responded, "Well, you know what they also say, you get what you pay for."

This time, however, I didn't laugh. And Sashima didn't look over to question why I was not laughing. We just sat in silence staring out into the ocean from our perches on the Pacific Beach boardwalk.

I didn't know how to respond to that comment. *What does that comment mean anyway?* I thought to myself. *You get what you pay for. What does it mean in this context?* I had no clue. All I knew is that it ended in a preposition so there must be more to it. Or perhaps it just needed to be re-worded. *You get that for which you pay. OK, sounds better and … I still don't know what it means in this context. But wait; let's try it on again. And this time, I'll pray the ACIM prayer. Holy Spirit, help me to see this differently. What does 'you get that for which you pay' mean in this context?*

46

"Sashima?" Hearing my own voice speak aloud rather than in my head startled me as much as my voice startled Sashima. She must have been deep in thought as well.

"There is no cost to being open to learn from all the teachers that walk into our life in every moment. We pay nothing. And we get everything."

Sashima sat in silence a moment longer and then looked over at me. I saw her smile out of the right corner of my eye so I looked away from the ocean and toward her, smiling back. The sparkle in her eyes let me know that she had no more questions. My teacher was satisfied with my responses. I had learned all that I needed to learn in that moment.

Looking back at the ocean I was beaming from the inside out. *Well that was another unexpected learning moment with an unexpected teacher. And it cost me nothing. I just needed to be awake enough to realize that a learning opportunity had presented itself. And then I needed to agree to participate in my learning moment by being open and surrendering to not knowing. This stuff is so stinkin' cool. I love it! Thank you Universe. Thank you God. Thank you Holy Spirit. And heck, just for good measure, thank you Jesus!*

CHAPTER TEN

Ignoring versus Accepting

"I am not in denial." I exclaimed fervently. "I am in a state I like to call ignoring. There is a big difference." I glanced up to look into my friend Trina's eyes to see if she at all appeared to be convinced by my defensive posture and edicts that were spewing from my mouth.

She didn't. Her face remained stern and she didn't even look down into her cup of tea. She just kept staring at me.

"Right," she said sarcastically. "And what exactly is the difference between denial and your so called state of ignoring?"

Excellent, I thought. *I know the answer to this question. And I do have an answer.*

"The difference is that ignoring is where you accept that you have to do something about something, you are just not choosing to act on it right now. Denial is refusing to face the condition at all." I beamed in satisfaction to my well-crafted response to her question. I was just so very proud of myself.

"Right," she responded again. And I couldn't help notice that the sarcasm in her voice had grown, as did the intensity of her gaze into my eyes. "So, how is ignoring different than denial in appearance? I mean, how would I tell by someone's actions that they were in a state of ignoring versus a state of denial? Or is the difference only apparent in their head?"

Damn, she is good. I glanced down at my cup of tea and then back towards the ocean. *I think I will get some more hot water in this soon. My tea bag looks like it could handle another refill.* Trina and I were sitting at one of my favorite thinking and talking spots on the boardwalk of Pacific Beach, right across from the Cantina. The sun was bright and warm on that spring day. There was no hint of the approaching "May grey" as we affectionately referred to in San Diego. As I looked out at the ocean, I was confident I could see clearly for miles and miles and miles. But that was what my physical eyes could see on this gorgeous spring morning. With regard to Trina's question? Well, I couldn't see my way out of the densely soaked tea bag that was now resting along side my empty cup.

"Wanna get a refill and then continue on our walk?" I cheerily asked Trina. She nodded slowly with a slight grin on her face and a knowing twinkle in her eye. She knew I wasn't able to answer her question and she was giving me a reprieve before returning to her inquiry.

We refilled our cups with hot water, took a moment to chit chat with some tourists, offering them advice on the must sees and dos in San Diego County before heading back south along the boardwalk to continue our beloved time together. We walked in silence for a while and then I spoke in an attempt to answer Trina's question.

"Thank you Trina. I hear what you are saying. I will return the phone calls and get the imaging scheduled and I will follow up with another consultation to the doctor. You are right. There is no difference in what the action of ignoring and denial look like. The non-action inherent in both looks exactly the same. I hear you, I hear you. It is time for me to move back into action. I will get it all scheduled."

I didn't make eye contact with Trina as I spoke. My gaze shifted between watching where my feet were landing on the boardwalk and watching the surfers challenge the waves in the ocean. *Man I am so lucky. I can't believe I get to live here.*

"Well, for what it is worth, you are funny. Your trying to explain that there is a difference between the state of ignoring and the state of denial was funny." Trina chided throwing her arm around my shoulders.

"Yes," I exclaimed in victory. *I so love it when someone thinks I am funny.*

"So, how is Leanna's mom doing?" Trina asked. The shift in topic was welcomed for me. Yet, this would also be painful. Leanna's mom's cancer had returned after an eleven-year remission. She was in ICU as she had gone into shock from the intense chemotherapy treatment they had administered after removing all of her small intestine. It was her first chemotherapy treatment after her surgery and it had gone horribly wrong. Leanna's mom had gotten deathly sick from the chemo. The doctor's had given up on any alternative for her. They didn't know what to do next for the treatment had left Leanna, her mom, and her dad reeling. Leanna's mom was tiny; down to 71 pounds. We were all more than concerned about Leanna, her dad, and her mom. Yet we were unsure how to best show up in love and support for all three of them.

As I brought Trina up-to-date on Leanna's mom, my phone rang. It was Edwardo, the man I had recently met and with whom I was already fully taken. Edwardo was a charmer and he was genuine, a deadly combination for me.

I excused myself from Trina to take the phone call and as I did, I noticed her smirk. I was definitely going to be teased about taking a phone call from a boy during sacred girl talk time. *Oh well, he is worth it.* I quickly spoke to Edwardo about finalizing our plans for that evening and then he took a moment longer to share his latest idea with me. It was brilliant and sharing it with me was perfect timing. I couldn't wait to share his idea with Trina. Finishing the call as graciously yet as quickly as I could, I returned my attention to Trina who was still, yes, smirking.

"Don't even start with me Trina. Yes, I like him. I like him. He is a good guy and yes, we are having fun. And no, I doubt I will be dating him a month from now but for now, it is good." The defensiveness in my voice only made Trina smile more broadly. So, I had to move quickly to distract her from what I didn't want to hear, which was more teasing about how I have no clue how to date properly. Thus, I shared with her Edwardo's idea to find a time where everyone could send positive thoughts and prayers to Leanna's mom. Our intention was to ask Leanna to pick a date and a time. And then we would send out an email to as many people as possible asking them to send Leanna and her mom all these positive thoughts and prayers while Leanna was holding her mom in that same moment. We intended to have these thoughts and prayers heal Leanna's mom enough so that she could be released from ICU and eventually be strong enough to seek alternative treatment at a soft tissue sarcoma center in L.A. Leanna's mom had such an adverse reaction to her very first chemotherapy that alternative treatment had to be sought. Giving up just didn't seem like the right option at all.

Trina loved the idea and we began to think about all the folks we could invite to participate. We took a moment more to call Leanna and share the idea with her so that she could find the perfect moment to be with her mom, holding her in great love and joy, while we sent all the healing thoughts and prayers her way. Leanna loved the idea and promised she would get back to us with a suggested date and time so that we could get the word out.

"Wow, that was pretty wild – huh?" Trina exclaimed when I hung up the phone with Leanna.

Perplexed by her comment, I asked her to explain what she meant.

"Well, we were initially talking about how you have been ignoring your health situation and then we talked about Leanna's mom and their need to accept that this set of doctor's they trusted has no more alternatives for them. So, we need to send positive thoughts her way so she can get strong enough to seek an alternative source of therapy."

Trina was summarizing our earlier conversation but I didn't follow the connection she was making. My face contorted in confusion and Trina smiled more broadly at the site of it all. Her eyes were twinkling.

"Yeah," I responded my face still contorted. "Yeah, that's pretty much the situation. What is so wild about it?" I inquired hungry to understand what I was not seeing.

Trina's eyes glistened as she responded, still smiling broadly. "I don't think it is a coincidence that when you moved from denial to acceptance that you were in denial, you got that phone call. I also don't think it is a coincidence that when you spoke with Leanna about another option for her mom to feel well enough to go see an alternate doctor for alternative treatment, that they were open to your suggestion. I mean they usually don't buy into the kind of stuff you were suggesting – right?"

"Yeah, right." I mumbled, still perplexed by the point that Trina was making.

"Acceptance expands energy; acceptance expands possibilities. Ignoring and denial closes down energy. You accepted that you were in denial and in so doing, energy expanded. We start talking about Leanna and her mom and Edwardo calls with a great idea about how to create even more positive, healing energy." Trina was glowing.

"Aw…." I slowly awakened to the meaning of what she was conveying. "Yes, you are brilliant Trina. There are no coincidences. It is all as it is and we can continue to participate in a manner that allows more energy to expand and therefore more opportunities to open, or we can choose not to do so and watch energy contract and possibilities diminish."

"Exactly," Trina announced in glorious triumph.

Upon hearing her joyful exclamation, I was half expecting to see a band of angels descend blowing their long shiny brass trumpets. Instead, about 6 low-flying sea gulls buzzed by, startling me. I became agitated with them and hollered out to them calling them flying rats. In return, the latent seventh sea gull buzzed by to join the six and gave me a gift of her poop… right on top of my teacup.

Trina burst into laughter. I looked down at my cup and back up at her.

"No coincidences," I repeated. And I shouted to the seventh sea gull in appreciation for reminding me how diverse energy expansion and contraction can be seen.

CHAPTER ELEVEN

Dating My Mirror

"Who do I always end up dating? I end up dating the person that is the mirror image of who I am being. When I was unavailable, I attracted men who were completely unavailable. When I just wanted fun, I attracted men who just wanted fun. When I wanted a committed relationship, I attracted men who wanted to propose to me within three days of meeting me. When I wasn't trying to attract anyone, I ran into men who were doing the same. It is true what they say – you attract that which you are being, not that which you are seeking. Therefore, I attract the one that reflects me; that reflects the way I am showing up in the world. Dating is just looking into one big ass mirror." I finished my speech and the voice on the other end of the phone was silent.

"Edwardo? Did you hear what I said?" In that moment, I realized I had gone off on a tangent. I spoke with a bit of panic into the phone wondering if he had fallen asleep or whether the call had dropped. I pulled my cell phone away from my ear and looked at it to check the number of bars. As I did so, I heard his voice and I quickly yanked the phone back to my ear with such force that I winced in pain as the corner of the I-phone hit my cheekbone. *Ow, that hurt.*

"I am here darling. What is it you are trying to say?" The moment I heard Edwardo's smooth and sultry voice, my panic eased and my heart melted a little more.

"I am trying to say that when I look at you, I see the pimple on my face. The more I relate to you, the pimple starts to grow. I hate my pimple. And furthermore, I blame the chocolate I ate for my pimple that continues to grow. When I turn away from you and ask my friends if they also see how obnoxious my pimple has become, they tell me that they can't even see the pimple. They have no idea what I am talking about. Does that make sense?" I could feel the level of panic rising once again in my voice. And I realized that this was so not a conversation that I should be having over the phone. I couldn't see Edwardo's beautiful brown eyes and I couldn't tell how he was taking in all of my rhetoric.

His soft and gentle voice came over the phone again, "I hear your words darling but I still don't know what you are trying to say."

I sighed a deep sigh and with the sigh, the tears began to fall. "I want to have a baby and I can't. I am angry that I can't have a baby. I know you want a baby Edwardo. When I look at you, I see a father, I see someone who would be a great father, and I can't give you the baby. I always thought I would have a little girl yet I can't give you or me that little girl. I am not angry with you; you get to still have a baby. You should go find someone to be with who can give you the little girl your heart has always desired."

"Are you breaking up with me?" his startled voice, yet still gentle and loving, shook me. His words stung my heart.

I paused before responding. "I am letting you go Edwardo. I am letting you go so you can find the woman you deserve who can give you the little girl you so badly desire. I love you so much. I don't want to keep you from your joy and your heart's desire." Tears were streaming down my cheeks. The tears were flowing so forcefully, they were settling onto my phone and then dripping onto the kitchen counter where I sat perched on my trusty kitchen barstool. I couldn't believe I was actually having this conversation with a man I love over a cell phone while seated at my kitchen counter.

There was silence on the other end of the phone. And then I heard him say once again, "Are you breaking up with me Marilee?"

This time I didn't pause. I felt I just had to get it out.

"Yes," I said feeling my heartache, yet believing in my head that this was absolutely the right thing to do. "Yes Edwardo. I want you to go date someone who is younger, sweeter, more innocent than me, someone who can give you your little girl."

"So, you are breaking up with me then?" He replied once more and I nodded in response, thinking he could actually see me. My silence did not detain him. "Well, I don't see how this all fits into the pimple story or the dating is a mirror thing."

His frank and gentle question caused me to burst into laughter. It was just what I needed to hear. It was just the perfect moment of inflection of humor. His humor had perfect timing. Along with the many things that I had come to adore about Edwardo, the timing of his humorous inflections was something that I had come to appreciate in him. I could sense that he was pleased that he got me to move from crying to laughing. And I began to try to explain things to him amidst moments of wiping my tears, blowing my nose, and giggling.

I explained to Edwardo that I felt I attracted him into my life because I wasn't looking for anyone. I was convinced I would no longer date. My life was so full and rich and I was filled with joy. While I wanted an intimate connection with a special someone, I was resigned to thinking that it just was not going to happen or at least not in the way I had perhaps originally envisioned. Edwardo listened patiently as I continued. I explained to him that he struck me as being in the same place in that he was not looking for anyone, he was just enjoying his friends and his life and then we just happened to meet and well, it was a great connection. He was my mirror as we were both so content; the contentment in the mirror made a powerful reflection and projection. And all that seemed to feed into what else I saw in him: compassion, generous expressions of heart-felt love, constant considerate acts of kindness, gentle expressions of wisdom, soul-filled conversations, acts of faith and love, as well as bold actions of conviction and integrity. I fell for him and learning of some of his dreams, they were mine as well. However, I could no longer have one of those dreams and he could. I wanted him to have his dream of having his little girl. And maybe if he got his dream, I would get mine by seeing the joy in him having his dream come true.

Edwardo just kept listening as I continued. The pimple, I explained, was my need to protect myself. It was my insane way that I over-managed everything in my life. I knew that as I was seeing him, I was seeing my pimple - my need to protect myself grow larger and larger. I was seeing that the more I was taken with him and the more I wanted to spend time with him, the larger the need to protect myself grew. Since I knew he wanted to have a child and I knew I couldn't, it just seemed like a good idea to break up with him before I became even more accustomed to having him in my life, before I discovered more things to love about him, before he realized that he did in fact need to have his little girl – the little girl I could not give to him. Yes, my friends thought I was insane.

"Why would you break up with someone you love because you think they won't want to be with you because you can't have a baby?" they exclaimed to me. They were telling me that it was not mine to break up with Edwardo; it was only mine to tell him the truth, which was the fact that I could no longer become fertile. And then it would be left up to him to decide what to do and most likely, we would have a conversation about it and then make a decision together about whether to continue to date. But no, I had to go and break up with him because the pimple on my face was getting larger and larger. I had to pop it; I just had to.

Edwardo listened, I could feel him listening intently and I was so grateful when he broke the silence. "I am glad I am not the pimple." I burst into laughter once again. *I love that he knows how to make me laugh.*

"Marilee, I am going to see you tomorrow. I know you just broke up with me and I know it is really late so I am not coming over tonight. But I am going to see you tomorrow. We will continue to discuss this then. I will call you in the morning to find a time that works well for you."

"OK," I responded relieved that I would get to see him again and grateful to him for holding such compassionate and non-judgmental space for me to express my fears and my understanding of why I do what I do. I thanked him, affirmed my love for him, and hung up the phone.

The tears began to flow again. Why did I feel so miserable if what I had done was so virtuous? Why did I feel so empty if what I had done was release a man I love to pursue his dreams? Wasn't that what love is all about anyway? Aren't we supposed to provide space for those we adore to be all they can be? If that is true, shouldn't I feel good about this?

I slid off my kitchen bar stool and made my way to the powder room to clean up my smeared mascara and lord only knows what else that was stuck on my face. As I peered into the delicate powder room mirror, I thought I saw a pimple. I leaned into the mirror and wiped away my clinging hair and mascara so that I could take a closer look. There was no pimple where I thought there had been. It looked however, like I had a bruise. I wondered, for a moment, if my pulling the phone back to my face with such force earlier in the evening caused what I saw on my face. Continuing to gaze into the mirror, I examined the mark further. Tears began to flow again when I realized that there was no pimple there, there was a bruise.

My need to over-manage my life, a relationship, a love, and a dream had once again caused a mark in my life. I may have popped the pimple and in so doing, I created a mark that looked even worse than the original pimple. After all it was a pimple and they sometimes go away on their own, particularly if you don't mess with them, if you don't pick at them. If you just let go of what feeds their growth, they often go away. Would this popped pimple, this mark turn into a scar or would it melt away? Time would tell, I guess. For now, I wasn't sure. All I knew is that I just needed to sit with this. I needed to be with this. I needed to let it alone and not pick at it. As I looked at it, I knew I would be reminded of the lesson learned and the choice that I had just made. I prayed that I would not make such a choice again in the future. But for now, I knew I needed to leave it be.

Backing away from the mirror and taking my stance of power, Tadasana, I announced with a pointed finger to the image in the powder room mirror.

"You will no longer over-manage your relationships. You will focus on being that which you were designed to be, and that is love. You are not fear. You are love. Fear manages; love does not. Just be love." I did my best to smile in the mirror and to look into my watery red eyes as I spoke. But my eyes kept glancing down at the spot where the mark appeared. *Was it getting bigger?* The tears returned.

As I backed out of the powder room and turned to go upstairs to my bedroom, my thoughts took over my heart. *I guess I just need to be with this for now. I just need to be in mourning over having made yet another decision out of fear even though I justified it as love. I just need to leave this mark alone and let it heal on its own. No picking! And I wonder what Edwardo will say to me tomorrow. Will he reflect my fear or will he choose love? It doesn't matter what Edwardo says; it doesn't matter what I see in his reflection tomorrow. What matters is that I get to choose again. And next time, I will choose love, real love, and true love, not fear justified as love.*

CHAPTER TWELVE

Preaching without Words

"I have simply had enough." I told my sister as we walked from the car to the super discount store to get much needed clothing, groceries, and toiletry items for our beloved relative and her children who were in dire need of someone to help them out in these wretched economic times.

"Enough of what?" my sister replied with the innocence that only she could have for someone who had experienced the hardship of life yet still remained so anchored in love. We had exited the rental car on this incredibly hot summer midwestern day. I had kept walking toward the store when she had stopped to ask me what I was talking about. My sister, Liza, was so full of love and presence that I often forgot that in moments like these, she would literally stop what she was doing, no matter how pressed for time she was to make sure that her full attention was on the one she wanted to understand. In this situation, I was the blessed one who had gained her attention.

Smiling warmly to myself after realizing that I had walked on forgetting her ability to be so present, I turned back around to face her. I grabbed her by the arm as if to signal that I was fine and well aware of our time crunch, pulled her arm lovingly into mine as if I was her escort and proceeded to move back toward the entrance of the store. Her hazel warm eyes sparkled in agreement as she moved with me yet repeated the question with more compassion than St. Francis himself could ever show even on his best day.

"Enough of what Marilee?"

"Enough of the lies." I replied and the sound of my own anger in my voice sent shivers down my own spine. I released Liza's arm so as to not have her feel my tremors. I hadn't realized how angry I was at the situation we found ourselves in until I heard myself speak in that moment.

She and I had taken off of work, spent money we really didn't have to check in on our parents, siblings, and their kids along with other relatives. These were the times where everyone was economically hurting regardless of how well off they had been in previous years. In particular, the toll of the economic hardship was showing up in some very specific situations. I had passed judgment as to why some were suffering more than others and I hadn't realized I had done that until just this moment.

My sister, the one with more compassion and tenderness than St. Francis himself, remained silent. When she spoke, I was surprised with the fact that she was pointing out the quote on my t-shirt instead of responding to the words I spoke.

"You know who said those words, don't you, Marilee?"

"What words? The words, 'I have had enough of the lies?' Was it Clint Eastwood in some shoot-'em-up movie?" I was still startled by the amount of anger in my voice.

Laughing at my very serious answer, she pointed to the words on my t-shirt, which read, *Preach all the time, sometimes even with words.* I had forgotten which t-shirt I was wearing in that moment and I was grateful she had pointed it out. For here I was in the mega super discount store parking lot ready to cuss up a storm about how frustrated I was with our family situation when I was wearing my Level I Baptiste Institute Yoga Boot Camp [17] survival t-shirt.

"Naw, I don't know who said these words." I announced looking down at the words on the front of my t-shirt. "The saying is in quotes

---

17   Baron Baptiste Power Vinyasa Yoga – www.baronbaptiste.com

but there is no citation. Holy Moses, I should have pointed that out to these folks. That is bad form; a quote with no proper citation. What kind of scholar am I anyway?"

Giggling even more, Liza rolled her eyes and replied.

"St Francis wrote it Marilee. That quote is from St. Francis."

Well of course she knows this. She and St. Francis gotta be tight. I mean she acts just like I hear he acted. Of course she knows that he wrote this quote. She is probably him re-incarnated, I mean, if there is such a thing as re-incarnation.

"Really?" I replied, all signs of anger now removed for how can you talk about St. Francis of Assisi and remain pissed off. "Fascinating. Thank you. I'll call the Baptiste people and make sure they give him the citation on any more t-shirts they print. Hey, I wonder if they now owe him royalties."

Laughing even harder, she spoke again.

"Come on Marilee. Time to preach without words." With that, we entered the super mega discount store, grabbed two carts, both unwieldy and wobbly as I have ever witnessed a shopping cart to be and proceeded to load up on items that our dear sweet relative desperately needed.

As we divided up the shopping list, I thought about my anger, my judgment of the situation, and my sister's wise reminder of the words I was wearing so boldly on my chest. I found myself in a tight spot on the fine line where I encouraged Tina to take care of her own needs but forgot to remind her to be mindful of the ramifications of those decisions that she made. I forgot to remind her that, as she tends to her own needs, she needs to consider the ramifications of her decisions on the community that surrounds her. In this situation, the community was Tina's own family and Tina's decision was to leave town in a time of crisis. I understood her decision. She needed to leave, her daughter's third pregnancy out of wedlock was too much for her to handle. And at the same time, the ramifications of that decision – the decision for Tina to up and leave town - left her family reeling, wondering what to do and where to go for help.

I was further exasperated because the origin of this crisis situation was veiled in lies. Nothing made sense and it appeared that we were never going to fully understand what had happened. All we knew was what we faced and the needs that seemed to be apparent. We were taking food and supplies over to Tina's daughter's, Stacie's apartment where her two children were with her, along with the third unborn child. Although quite frankly, I wasn't even sure we were reading the needs accurately. No one wanted to discuss what had really happened with Tina leaving town suddenly and Stacie's horrifying auto accident. No one wanted to answer the questions of how we had all come to be in the situation that led us to the super mega discount store. I felt my anger stir again within my chest.

Why was I angry? I was angry because I didn't know the truth of the current situation or the truth of what had led to the creation of the current situation. All I knew was that we had Stacie with a 5 year old, a 2 year old, and an unborn child who had survived a horrendous car crash. They were in need of the basics and no one seemed to give a shit about it at all. And just a few hours earlier, I had been in conversation with the group of relatives where I felt like I couldn't do anything about it at all either. So what changed? My sister Liza telling me that I was not allowed to stand by and watch this or even ignore it. I was in town for 18 more hours and by god, I was going to do something about it along with her.

I resisted at first explaining that my help was never appreciated or even welcomed in that family – the family whose needs now led us to our shopping spree in the super mega discount store. Previously, anytime I tried to get folks in that family to question the situation in which they found themselves, and inquire into what role they had in getting themselves in that situation, I was called a woman libber, a radical Liberal, and someone who tore up happy homes for a reason I actually never had the opportunity to hear. Regardless of what I was called or labeled, their strategy worked and I found myself staying on the outside looking in at the heartache, just watching, sending up prayers, and never doing anything more than hoping for turnarounds in their lives where more love, joy, and peace would flow more freely.

Well, today was different because Liza reminded me that the strategy only had worked because I had become concerned about not looking like any of the names I had been called. I had in some sort of distorted way believed that what these folks who didn't want me to ask them questions and get them to ask questions of their own situations had said about me. My concern for looking good or not wanting to look like the names that this family had called me kept me from preaching without words.

As we loaded our two cartloads of gifts into the rental car – my purchases were placed in the trunk and hers in the back seat – we slid into the overheated car with great discomfort and without speaking. We were trying not to burn our bare legs on the hot dark upholstery. Finally, Liza, asked me, "How is your dissonance resolving itself?"

I must digress here for a moment. Liza, along with several of my friends decided that asking someone how they are is just about the most insincere question you could ask anyone ever. What we mean by that is that if you know the least bit about what is going on in a loved one's life, you will be asking them about that...not something as disingenuous as "how are you?" What does that really ask anyway, especially in the United States. Heck, here, that is the same as saying, "Hello," or "Hey there," or "oh my gosh, I ran into you and I know you and I have to say something to you or else you will think me rude so I'll just say how are you?" If you really care about someone and how they are doing, ask them something specific pertaining to their life. And that is exactly what Liza was doing in this moment when she asked me how my dissonance was resolving itself. What a beautiful question. So I responded.

"My anger is still present. I am still finding myself in judgment of a situation that seems to have been caused by patterns of neglect. I feel caught in a cycle of judgment and I know that if I stay there, I won't be showing up in love and in a space where the Holy Spirit can work through me to be love and to be with them in their pain." I felt as if I was rambling and I felt I was in confession. But what I felt was genuine. It was real. I had decided to quit pretending in order to appear loving.

Instead, I had decided to be with all that I was feeling. It didn't feel good, but it felt very real and very genuine and that felt freeing.

Liza paused and just started the car long enough to roll down the electric windows to allow for cooling air to flow before shutting the car off once again. She shifted her legs with a grimace as if to denote the hot upholstery had caught a corner of her hand burning it slightly before she could lift it back away from the car seat. She sat in silence a moment longer as if seeking divine wisdom before she spoke.

"If you knew the truth of this situation and if you knew the truth of what led up to it, would you be doing anything differently right now in this moment?"

Damn good question. "I don't know Liza. I really don't. Perhaps. Perhaps, I would be at the father of Stacie's children's home giving him a lecture about showing up in responsibility for her and his offspring. Perhaps I would be at her sister's or her father's giving the same lecture. Perhaps, I would be sending out the police after Tina to track her down and tell her to get her ass back into town. I don't know. I just don't know."

Liza sighed and shifted back to face the steering wheel, this time without a grimace of pain. I thought she was going to start the car again but instead she reached for the door knob, opened the car door and got fully out of the car, shutting the door behind her, windows still fully open.

"Liza, where are you going?" I asked completely bewildered by her actions.

She leaned forward with her head and chest framed by the car door window and arms carefully away from the car so as to not get burned by the radiating heat from outside of the car door.

"Marilee, if you need understanding of this situation in order to contribute to providing for the basic needs of the children involved in this situation, then I recommend you return all the items you bought. I am opening the trunk to help you return the gifts you purchased." With that she stood straight up, and moved to the back of the car to open the trunk.

Bewildered even more and in a bit of a panic, I threw open my car door almost hitting the car door next to me. Frantically, I scurried out of my seat, almost falling to the ground to get to the back of the car where Liza stood peering over the purchases I had made.

"No, no, no" I yelled at Liza. "No, the gifts for the children stay. The gifts for the children stay. They didn't choose to be in this situation."

"Exactly," Liza said as she slammed the trunk lid with such force that it sent me falling backwards behind it. "Get back in the car Marilee. We have a delivery to make."

I did as Liza advised. I slid back into the car and we drove to Stacie's apartment without further comment. I was thinking about preaching without words and I was thinking about judgment. I was thinking about how my advice to this family had fallen on ears that wouldn't listen and I was thinking of all the hurtful things that they had said about me and to me because I had tried to help them by using my words. And now, in this moment, Liza's actions had helped me understand the true meaning of preaching without words. This was not a time to understand, this was not a time to seek the truth of the situation or of that, which led to the creation of the situation. This was not a time to get everyone to think about his or her role in making this all happen. This was a time to take care of the little ones who didn't choose to be in this situation, who had nothing to do with its creation.

There was no doubt in my mind as we drove to that apartment that the time for words would come. The time for seeking the truth would come. The time for responsibility for actions and understanding the ramifications of individual actions would take place. For now, however, it was time for no words to be spoken. There were mouths to be fed, and bodies to be nurtured, healed, and clothed. It was time for love in action.

CHAPTER THIRTEEN

Finding the Right Question

I glanced out the window of my hotel room one more time to see all the folks lining up to go to the play-off game. I had the most perfect view of entry number 8 to Roger's Arena from my hotel room. I was in Vancouver, British Columbia, a gorgeous city. I had the privilege of being there to work on some research with a few other university partners from other countries and our second day of meetings had ended early to get out of the way for the Canuck's play-off game; they were competing for the Stanley Cup.

I really wanted to go to the game but I knew I had a ton of work to do plus, I really didn't have the money that would be required to buy a scalped ticket. But believe me, I really thought about what I could go without in order to get a seat in that arena. Instead of looking for a scalped ticket, I was fully enjoying the joyous noises arising from the streets as I sat at my desk to read my email.

Glancing from my hotel room perch from above the crowds on the street, I looked back down at my laptop with a big smile on my face. I saw an email from a colleague who had become a dear friend and with whom I had not spoken to in several years. It read:

Hello Marilee,

I know it has been a long time since I emailed you. I always appreciate your emails and the updates on your life and health and I am hoping that things are going reasonably well for you.

I had to clean out my office in the last few days as we are moving here and I came across a card you had given me a long time ago. It made me very nostalgic and made me remember the good old times.

There is something I had been meaning to ask you all these years because I always wondered why you had said or written it to me at the time, but I never quite found the courage to ask you. Although I don't quite remember the context, a long time ago you said something to me along the lines that "if Allen ever hurt me, I should let you know", and I have always wondered in all these years why you said this and whether you said this to me because you knew something about him that I was blind to.

Allen and I are still together and we surely had and still have our ups and downs. He had been going through some extremely rough times during his PhD work and life was pretty brutal for both of us at the time. I do think that he loves me very much, but I also think that just being with me is not enough for him. He has hurt me quite badly over the years, and although I am only aware of one affair he had, I would not be surprised if there were several others. Sadly, he never had the courage to admit any of these things (apart from the one occasion where I more or less caught him) and that makes it difficult for me to try to help find a solution that we can both be happy with. I love him very much and I wish sometimes I could just close my eyes and be blind to all these things, but sometimes I have moments where I feel that I can't handle the pain anymore. I want to understand where this drive comes from and why he is doing this, but any upfront communications seems rather difficult because unless I start snooping behind his back, he will not be open to talk about it. So, I am just trying on my own now, without invading his privacy, to find some clues and understand better what has really been going on in all these years. And maybe all these thoughts are just ghosts in my brain, that is of course a possibility also. Maybe these other occurrences were very harmless and I am just simply over-reacting. Maybe I am completely off base here, and I hope you understand that I am not trying to imply anything here that has anything to do with you. I just had this thought for many years now and simply just wondered why you said this to me and I finally found the courage to ask.

Of course, Allen does not know that I am searching for some explanations and therefore I of course would greatly appreciate it if you would keep this email confidential. If you want to talk rather than email, feel free to call me at work. My direct number is listed in the signature line below. Again, I hope you won't take this personal and if you just said it as a friend with no real reason behind it, then I won't wonder any longer.

I know one way or another, everything will be well in the end. I am hoping from the bottom of my heart that I can find a way to have him open up to me and help us find a solution together. Or have my brain once and for all cleared of these ugly thoughts and just find happiness together.

I really really appreciate your friendship and I hope to hear from you soon.

Take care

Sabrina

Holy Moses! Now that 'aint an email that I get every day. I wonder what happened to cause her to send this email now and to me? What had Allen done now? And what is she so afraid of? And why to me? What did my card say that she found in her office? Weird. Were my intentions that I was sending to the Universe to be loving and to help women step into their power being answered so quickly? How cool is that? And yet, how full of pain is Sabrina? Ooh, I can feel it. Holy Moses.

Glancing one more time over my left shoulder at the stadium, I saw the crowds growing in size and energy. I loved the excitement that was resonating from the street. I considered walking the short walk to the stadium to see if I could scalp a ticket for less than a hundred bucks. It would be so much fun to be in there watching the game. And then I thought again. It was not the amount of money that was keeping me from grabbing my jacket and venturing out of my hotel room, it was not the thought of wondering whether I could be thrown in the Canadian jail if I got caught for scalping a ticket (why is it legal for Stub Hub to do this and illegal for any Joe on the street anyway – that makes NO sense to me). It was the pain in Sabrina's email that kept me leashed to my desk. I wanted to answer it if I could.

So, I re-focused my attention on my laptop and re-read Sabrina's email. I could feel her pain and I could feel her fear. I prayed for guidance and I responded.

Dearest Sabrina,

It is so wonderful to hear from you. I miss you so very much! You are such a beautiful soul and I consider it such an honor to have you in my life.

You can ask me anything anytime. I am here for you.

Here are some things to consider in your inquiry process.

You most likely know the answer to the question you are asking so perhaps you are not searching for the answer but searching for a way to accept the answer that you already know to be true.

There has never been any doubt in my mind that you love Allen and that Allen loves you. What I wondered when I asked you that question, so many years ago, was whether the way that Allen loves you would be the way that you wanted to be loved. Would the way that Allen loves you cause you pain? What I mean by this is that, for example, I have no room for the man to whom I am committed to physically engage in intercourse with another woman. I don't get jealous, I am simply intolerant. He has to physically love me and only me. If he has lustful eyes for others, he better be really good at not letting me ever find out – not even a clue. Yet, when I have loved men that are not able to physically love only me, I always found out. At first, I needed proof, even though I just knew. Now, I don't need proof. I trust my sense of knowing. (After all, we women are superior with that kind of thing. LOL.) When I discovered this about my man – that he physically loved more than just me - that doesn't mean that I didn't love my man or that he didn't love me. I knew that he did. It just meant that I have one way that I preferred to be loved and that he may have another way to love. Does that make sense? So given all this...

How do you want to be loved? And why do you feel that you have to justify how you want to be loved or how you expect to be loved? Would you be open to just stating to Allen what you expect from him as your lover and then give him the opportunity to determine, without judgment from you, whether he can meet your expectations? That way, the burden of finding out the truth or the burden of understanding him is removed from you and placed where it belongs...on him. My friend Cathy often reminds me that when I misunderstand a man I am dating or he misunderstands me, the best way to clear up the misunderstanding is to focus on explaining what I understand about myself rather than telling him what I understand about him. In that way, I remain removed from judging him through my eyes and remain more focused on what I know – which is me and how I feel. Similarly, if I don't understand something that he does, it is his to explain or mine to let go of, not mine to figure out. It may sound weird, but it is really freeing in that I am not taking responsibility for what is not mine. Basically, his job is to know himself and speak his needs and desires. My job is to know myself and speak my needs and desires. Together, we listen without judgment as we genuinely share with each other how we can remain authentic and address each other's stated needs and desires or how we cannot.

Maybe it would be good for me to share a specific example here. I very much love Tony, the man I met on my way to interview for the job at San Diego State about 6 years ago. As a matter of fact, I am in Vancouver now and I just texted him sincerely that I wish he were here to go to the Canucks hockey game tonight with me. (He loves hockey and I know he will be watching the game on television tonight.) I love Tony and I know Tony loves me however Tony is not, nor ever will be a "one woman kind of guy". He is always there for me when I need him and we chat a lot. However, Tony is not able to physically love only one woman at a time. I had so many heartaches on the road to discovering this truth. And I spent so much energy trying to understand him and how he works and why this is so, blah, blah, blah… In the end, I realized that Tony is just not made that way. He would get angry with me every time I got hurt over something he did that reminded me of this truth. I could either accept that he is this way and keep him as my lover or I could say, that is so not what I want. The option to expect him to change was never really a viable option. It was just another expectation I placed on him that made him angry. I chose to tell Tony that he is not what I want. He wanted me to so badly accept him for what he is and to be fine with how things are but that is not what I wanted. I just don't want that kind of partner in my life. I don't judge him for it but I judged me for wanting something different – after all I did love him and I adore him. It took me a while to accept Tony's way of being as a truth about him and quite frankly now, I could care less whether he accepts it about himself. However for a while, that was not the case. I kept wanting him to explain why he was this way to me and I kept needing to understand, blah, blah, blah. Then I realized that my bigger step was accepting that I didn't want that in my life – that it was OK for me to want something other than what Tony is or is not. What is important now is that I know what I want and it is not that. What I want in a partner is not to be confused with whether I love Tony or he loves me. We do love each other; this way of loving each other is just not what I want to experience in a committed relationship.

So my gorgeous Sabrina, from where I sit, you can either continue on your investigation of Allen's choices, trying to understand why he is the way he is or you can decide that what you already know is enough. If you choose the latter, than you can decide whether this will be something you can accept about him or not.

I feel that love is all encompassing; it means we accept everything about someone for what it is and what it is not. We accept all that they are for who they are and who they are not. But it doesn't mean that we have to live with that. It is much easier for me to love Tony as everything he is and is not now because I am not considering him as a partner. We are much better friends now than we ever were as lovers. Yes, I would like to spend more time with him than I do. And even though he is dating someone else, he still wants to sleep with me and I say no. He hasn't changed. I don't want that in my life as a lover, as a partner, but I can take him fully as a friend.

I recently took some time to write about what it is that I think love is for me; and what it looks like and feels like. I encourage you to do the same. Maybe you will see Allen in what you write and maybe you won't. In any event, it may help you feel better about the choices you want to make. It may empower you to know that you deserve that which you want and that which you don't want. And it then may empower you to choose that which you want and that which you don't want.

In love and in light,

Marilee

Pushing my chair back away from my desk, I glanced over my left shoulder towards Roger's arena, more blue and green – the Canuck's colors – were spotting the walkway of entrance number 8. The joy that I felt from this scene seemed in direct conflict to the sorrow that was on my laptop before me.

Life is so weird I thought to myself. The people there on the streets below are celebrating a competition and expecting a forthcoming victory. The woman whose email lies before me is across the continent and in pain, wondering why she can't understand how it is that the "love of her life" is who he is loving her in the way he does or does not. I glanced down at the clock ticking away on the hotel room desk, wondering if I should try to make it to the game. I still had time; I could make it if I ran. But then I realized I most likely did not have enough cash in my wallet to buy a scalped ticket. And I didn't really want to run. I wanted to re-read my email to Sabrina and send it off to her, praying that it would bring her some sort of semblance of comfort; praying she would find the questions that made sense for her to ask and the answers that would lead her closer to discovering peace.

Life is so weird. It is joy and pain and celebrations and mourning. And I guess it can all be made so much more tolerable when we ask the questions that we need to ask and when we accept what is and what is not. And it can be made so much more joyful when we move within the flow of that acceptance, ask different questions, and discover answers that can make a difference. Is that thought anything like Wayne Gretzky's [18] analogy of skating to where the puck is going versus where it is? *Holy shit, it is.* When I accept what is and isn't, I can skate to where the puck is going - to where the energy is flowing because I am no longer resisting seeing what is and what is not. I am no longer just focused on what is but what is becoming. *Cool!*

With that, I pressed the send button on the email to Sabrina, grabbed my jacket and whatever money I had in my wallet, and sprinted out the door to see if I could snag a ticket to the playoff game that was starting in 10 minutes. Go Canucks!

---

18   "I skate to where the puck is going to be, not where it has been."– Wayne Gretzky - http://www.brainyquote.com/quotes/authors/w/wayne_gretzky. html

CHAPTER FOURTEEN

Within Me

"You want the whole story?" I asked, my body still shaking from head to toe and the tears were still streaming down my face. I could tell from the sound of my voice that my body wasn't the only thing shaking, my voice was as well." But the 5'7" male police officer that answered my non-emergency phone call at 11:00 p.m. on a weekday night was as solid and unwavering as the pillar upon which I was leaning in my home.

"Well, what happened was I got home late last night from being out of town for 6 days. So, I had a lot of catching up to do. I was folding my clothes that I had just washed and dried on my bed in my master bedroom and I dropped a pillowcase on the floor by my headboard. For some reason, I was folding laundry on the side of bed that I don't sleep on; I don't really know why. I just was. In any event, as I bent over to pick up the pillowcase that I had dropped on the floor, I noticed something underneath my bed. It was a plastic tub - like the kind that you store sweaters in. I leaned down further and positioned myself to reach under the bed to pull it out to see what was inside. I had no idea how it had gotten there. It was just two weeks earlier when I had pulled the dining room table leaf from underneath my bed and returned it that same day because I had cooked dinner for a friend and her family who were in desperate need of cheer. That tub was definitely not under the bed then."

I had to stop to breathe. Police officer Gonzales was calm and patient while I caught my breath and continued.

"Well, I pulled that tub out and I looked inside of it and I freaked out. There was a black pair of Harley Davidson gloves, a black full-face ski cap, a black turtleneck, and black long underwear pants. I freaked. What the hell was that doing underneath my bed in my bedroom? I called a couple of friends thinking that they were trying to play some stupid freaky joke on me but they both denied it was theirs and encouraged me to call the police right away. That is where you come in; I am freaking out here. Who would do such a thing?" With that, I broke down into sobs again and clasped my face in my hands. I felt violated and thoughts of what could have happened to me in my home took over my mind. My body was shaking uncontrollably now and the sobs were loud and dramatic at best.

Officer Gonzales waited a moment for me to regain composure before he asked me questions that led me to explain to him that just about 9 days prior to this, a water valve had broken in my home and flooded the first floor, down to the garage. I had a couple of lock boxes on my home as contractors and restoration folks worked to bring my home back to its original condition. I didn't know if one of them had done this or if someone else had sneaked into the home and planted the box there while they were working. I didn't know. I didn't care. I just wanted the box out of my home, I wanted an investigation to begin, and I wanted the intruder shot in the groin. I think those were my exact words to Officer Gonzales anyway, but I am not quite sure.

Officer Gonzales explained to me that he couldn't do any of that. He explained to me that no crime had actually been committed.

"What?" I screamed out so loudly that the once solid as a pillar officer was now moved from his firm foundation. "You are telling me that there is no crime in some crazy asshole planting this box of black clothing underneath my bed, the bed I sleep in at night? You better be kidding me."

"Ma'am, I am not kidding you." He responded calmly and confidently. "The most you have here is trespassing."

"Trespassing? Are you fucking kidding me? Pardon my English. *I can't believe I just asked a police officer to forgive that I cussed right now. Holy Moses!* Seriously… someone entered my home, came into my bedroom, and placed black clothing underneath my bed. And all you can slap them with if you even find out who it is is trespassing? You gotta be fucking kidding me." And this time, I didn't apologize for my crass language.

Officer Gonzales patiently explained to me that since I had a lock box on my home, I had in essence given permission to folks I don't know to enter my property. I quickly countered with the explanation that there was no work to be done in my bedroom and entering my home to repair the flood damage did not mean I gave permission to them to either stage a robbery of one of my neighbors or rape me. There was no way this couldn't be a crime; intent was written all over that box. I could not believe what I was hearing from Officer Gonzales.

After several more minutes of him explaining to me what he could and could not do, I lost it. My tears had turned into anger and I gave poor Officer Gonzales a treatise he most likely did not deserve. I told him that this was exactly what was wrong with the law of the land. Someone has the right to harass a woman in all sorts of psychological and physical ways but there is nothing she could do about it to prevent further abuse. It wasn't a crime until she was killed. Or clearly they had planned to rob one of my neighbors and I had found compelling evidence of intent but they couldn't do anything about it until the crime had been committed.

"Unbelievable. Unfucking believable." I exclaimed to myself as Officer Gonzales left with the box of evidence. Shortly after he left, my friends Teresa and Raymond came over to stay the night with me. I was so grateful to see them when they rang the doorbell that I broke into tears again as I embraced them. I explained the events of the evening and ended with an angry tone as I told them how I had been made to feel helpless to take action, all because I trusted some contractors and restoration people by allowing them to put a lock box on my home to do a job that I would be paying good money for them to do.

Teresa and Raymond comforted me in their loving compassionate way, but my anger had now taken hold of me.

"I swear you guys. This is why people take the law into their own hands. Can you believe that? Can you believe that is not a crime? I didn't give permission to anyone to come into my bedroom, let alone plant a box of black clothing to use for robbery or rape or both. What is fucking wrong with the world?"

Teresa and Raymond just held me as I cried and vented. They sat in silence and in love. They didn't try to fix anything; they were just fully there. It was exactly what I needed.

After a long while of venting that led to saying some prayers of cleansing and protection, Teresa and I placed a statue of Buddha underneath my bed where the box had been. We wrote a sign to place by the Buddha that read, "Choose Love." Teresa prayed a prayer that was to remind me to fight evil with love and to remind me that love was more powerful than anything in the world. She reminded me of the ACIM teaching that everything is love or else it is a cry for love and she smiled from her heart as she did this. I could tell she really believed what she was praying. In that moment, I didn't believe a word she said. I heard the words but I didn't believe them. I was instead, still feeling violated and angry.

As Teresa and Raymond double checked to be sure I was alright, Teresa encouraged me to do an Angel Card [19] reading just before I slid off to sleep. I assured her I would and I closed the door to my bedroom and stood in the middle of my room facing the door feeling empty and disheartened. Do I really believe in the power of love? Do I feel strong at all? Do I feel weak and vulnerable and afraid? Or do I just feel angry and want to get a gun and shoot the bastard in the groin - the one who planted that tub underneath my bed? *Yup, I want to shoot the bastard in the groin. And then I want to drag the intruder's sorry ass down to the City Police*

---

19   Virtue, Doreen (2004). Archangel Oracle Cards. Carlsbad, CA: HayHouse Publishing.

Department, dump him at the feet of Officer Gonzales and say to the Officer, this man did not have permission to harass me so book him.

I stood in front of my bedroom door for a while. I wasn't sure I had the strength or the courage to turn and walk toward my bed. Yet, breathing deeply and intentionally, I found the strength. As I turned to face my bed, I remembered my promise to Teresa and I pulled the Angel cards from their drawer.

The Angel Cards were a gift from Teresa. The intent of the cards was to serve as an intercessory in times when I was troubled and unable to choose to listen to the Holy Spirit's guidance. Having come to believe that God speaks to everyone if we only are willing to listen, I no longer believed in the need for intercessors such as the priests that I had been raised to depend on for interpretation of God's word. I had come to believe that we all have been given the gift of the Holy Spirit which is the Spirit that helps us hear and interpret the word of God or will of God or path of God or whatever your religion calls it. I truly believe that there is one God for all religions, we just can't agree on what to name Him or Her and we certainly can't agree on how to interpret God's teachings. There seemed to be plenty of evidence to me that we all had the ability to interpret and that some of us – just as in our daily lives – were better listeners than others. So thus, some of us were better interpreters of what it all meant for the greater good than others. In this moment, I couldn't listen. I had fallen into the category of, "I ain't listening at all; and ain't willing to neither." Thus, the need for the Angel Cards; the need for an intercessory interpreter was absolutely necessary.

As I pulled out the Angel Cards from their deck, I knew I needed intercession. My anger was blocking the flow of all positive energy. I couldn't see peace, I couldn't feel love, and I wasn't sure what I believed. I prayed for the Archangels to present me with a message that they felt I most needed to hear in this moment and then I closed my eyes and drew a card. I paused for a moment before opening my eyes to read the card. I had to hold the card a moment longer and do my very best to choose to believe in the power of love. I didn't feel loving at all in that moment, but I chose to speak the words, "I choose love." Before opening my eyes.

When I opened my eyes, they fell upon the card that read, "Take Back Your Power; Use your God-given power and intention to manifest blessings in your life."

"Yes, I exclaimed aloud. "Yes!"

My enthusiastic announcement brought Teresa running out of her guest room located down the hallway. She flung open my closed door and ran into my bedroom. Teresa rushed over to where I sat on the floor, crouched over my Angel card. She was bending over to touch me and she spoke with a frightened, out-of-breath voice.

"What? What happened Marilee? Are you OK?"

Smiling for the first time in what felt like days, I looked up at Teresa and thanked her for her wisdom in advising me to do an Angel Card reading.

"Look what I pulled out," I exclaimed to her waving the card in front of her as if I was teasing her with her favorite kind of chocolate.

She enthusiastically pulled the card out of my hands, read it, glanced back at me, read it again, and visibly shivered in front of me. She closed her eyes and I felt her prayer of gratitude to the Archangels. I joined her in that prayer.

"Yes," I said aloud again and again, "thank you." I was still experiencing a moment of silent gratitude and joy when Teresa startled me with her enthusiasm.

"This is perfect. This is the greatest. I am so glad I came back in here to see this. I feel awesome, don't you?"

"Well…", I slowly began, my eyebrows wrinkling with concentration in trying to sense how I truly felt. "I still feel far from awesome but this is a damn good start." We both giggled as I stood up to meet Teresa. We embraced.

"Thank you Teresa. I will sleep beautifully well now."

We spent a moment longer to recap the miracle that had just transpired, checked under the bed to make sure that Buddha was still there (*why we did that, I have no idea…*) and hugged each other again wishing each other a warm and loving good night.

As Teresa left my bedroom with a gorgeous wide smile and a spring in her step, I lifted the card to read it one more time. "Take Back Your Power; Use your God-given power and intention to manifest blessings in your life."

Had I manifested this event? Had I become so off of center that I was creating all the chaos I was recently experiencing in my life? I was too tired to think anymore. I placed the card on my nightstand, glanced at it one more time, offered up a prayer of deep gratitude for my safety, for my friends, Teresa and Raymond, for the Archangel message, and for a warm and comfortable bed. It would be a night of restorative sleep.

Two evenings after the night that the box of black clothing was found underneath my bed, Teresa phoned to check in on me once again. She and my other priceless friends had been dutifully keeping an eye on my well-being. I was doing my best to make sure that this event wasn't dropping me back into past memories that I no longer wanted to recall. I felt that everyone's prayers were working beautifully. Yet, I was still wondering what role I had played in manifesting this event into my life.

After Teresa and I spoke briefly to simply catch up on each other's days, I asked her what she thought about my role in manifesting this event.

"You had no part in it Marilee. Don't do that to yourself." She responded rather emphatically.

"Thank you for your encouragement Teresa. I am grateful to you but honestly, I know I am walking off-of-center and I have been for a while. I can feel it."

Teresa's silence gave me all the affirmation I needed and she spoke with more of it.

"Yes Marilee, you have been off-of-center. I can see it. I have wanted to address this observation with you for a while but we have both been so very busy. There hasn't been any time." Teresa was always so thoughtful about when she brought up her accountability conversations. She always waited to be one-on-one with you when no one was around. I wasn't as sensitive. I would tell someone what I was seeing pretty much in any environment in front of well, pretty much anyone. It was something my friends had asked me to work on - - the whole being more discrete with what I observed and I had a long journey yet to walk.

I thanked Teresa for bringing forth her observations. Being the gorgeously accountable friend that she is, she made time right then and there to tell me more. We talked about how she had seen my energy appear scrambled and directionless. She had shared that she saw it begin when Garrison (see Rushing to Yoga) called off the engagement and that she had felt my scattered energy was rapidly increasing and that it was as scattered as she had seen it in recent weeks.

I had to agree with her. My meditation times were totally sucky. I couldn't sit in meditation well at all. I had sensed increasing agitation in areas that I thought I had "conquered" already such as driving in Southern California traffic. And I had also noticed that in my increasing desire to surrender, it seemed I was managing more situations at an increasingly high level of ridiculousness. When I was with Garrison, I could see love reflected in him to me. I never questioned the power of love when I was with him.

Now, I had to admit that I did. I hated to admit that. In my attempt to surrender, I felt I was actually trying to manage my life even more. It felt as if in seeking to manage more of my life, more chaos in my life was being created. I re-capped to Teresa that in the last three weeks, there had been an escalation in insanity in my life… the break-up with Edwardo, Taylor's stalking of me in my workplace, Tina's taking off unannounced when I flew into visit her and no one knowing where she went, Stacie's car accident when I went to see her and how she was with child when it happened and she also had her two daughters with her as well, the home flood, the increased pain caused by the aggressive endometrium growths which now meant 24/7 pain suppressors, Garrison's sudden loss of his hearing causing him to lose his job, my father's hospitalization, my increasing missing of work deadlines, the folks at work getting weird undiagnosable illnesses, my boss's husband losing his job unexpectedly, and the recent box of clothing underneath my bed… it was crazy. I felt as if

I was caught in a cyclone and I was very far away from the peace of its center.

"Something within me is contributing to this insanity Teresa. Either that or I am getting tested as to how much I truly am willing to surrender. What do you think?"

"I think, you need to pray on that Marilee. And I will too. We'll chat more later. I really need to run now. I'll be late meeting Raymond and Loretta for the concert if I don't get moving."

I thanked Teresa and hung up the phone. I always loved how much clarity came to me as I spoke with her. She really had a gift and I felt so fortunate to have her, along with the many other Angels who walked with me each day. I felt truly loved.

I feel truly loved. Do I really? Or am I just saying that right now because I should feel truly love.

"Quit shoulding on yourself Marilee." The voice of my sister who I had had the privilege of visiting the weekend prior to this most recent insanity came flooding to my ears and I giggled to myself as I placed the phone down on my kitchen counter.

"Yeah, Marilee, quit shoulding on yourself." I echoed allowed in my empty kitchen that was still being put back together from the flood. I looked around the empty dis-assembled kitchen and felt guilty for feeling sorry for myself. I had a home that could be repaired. There were so many folks with the recent tragedies in the south and in Japan who had no hope of ever getting their home restored. I shouldn't be feeling sorry for myself at all. *I am so blessed. I am so loved.*

"Quit shoulding on yourself Marilee." The voice of my sister came back to me again, but this time, I didn't giggle. Instead, I turned around, strode out of the kitchen and walked onto my stone patio. I laid down on the stone that my sister and my father had laid before he got sick. I took the pose of Savasana, sweet surrender.

I surrender to the uncertainty I feel within me. I surrender to not really knowing in this moment if I believe in the power of love. I surrender to the insanity that my being off center has created in my life. I surrender to not knowing how to fix it. I surrender to being angry with myself for being impatient with people I love, for feeling sorry for myself when I have no reason to, for being so behind at work, for missing my meditation and missing yoga classes…and well, just about everything. I surrender to this feeling of loss. I surrender to being completely confused and directionless. I just fucking surrender.

I repeated my surrender mantras and pledges a few more times. The last time I stated my surrender pledges in my head, I left out the cuss words. I closed my eyes and felt the setting sun kiss my face. It was a sweet kiss and I felt loved.

I feel love. I really feel love. I sat up suddenly almost bumping my head on my iron patio table. Giggling to myself I realized what I had been doing. I had lost the foundation of love that I had felt Garrison provided for me. In losing the foundation of love that Garrison had provided which was truly nothing more than Garrison's willingness to reflect my love back to me ('cause he always said that was just what he was doing), I had forgotten to love myself. I mean, I had done plenty of loving things for myself. I had gone on spiritual retreats, read inspirational passages, bought myself massages, pedicures, music, and spent time with people I loved. I had done plenty of things that nurtured my soul. I had engaged in acts of love toward myself, but they were empty because I forgot to simply be love. I had forgotten to simply be love and in so doing, I had failed to love me.

That is why I had lost faith in the power of love. I had remembered to engage in loving acts but I had forgotten to be love. Thus, my loving acts were empty, my energy was directionless. My energy was flowing out of control for the source of my being – that of love – was not present. I was co-creating this chaos because I had forgotten who I am…I had forgotten that as a child of God, I am love.

Excited to have been led to this discovery, I jumped to my feet. As quickly as I had jumped to my feet with this inspiring thought, I sat back down in defeat on the iron table that my head had nearly hit moments before. *How do I be love? I know how to engage in loving acts, but how do I be love? I have no frickin' clue.*

Glancing back down on the stone patio, I considered laying back down in Savasana and praying for more enlightenment, however the setting sun had made the stone cold and I was beginning to chill so I walked inside my home that was being restored. *How do I be love? I don't know. But I think I will begin by looking in the mirror and telling myself that I love myself for I am a child of God and I love God. Then I will continue with looking into the mirror and telling myself that I believe in the power of love. And then…well, I'll simply practice being present in every moment and when I forget to do that, I'll simply choose again in the next moment. And oh, yeah, I'll quit shoulding on myself too.*

I walked up the stairs to the powder room, turned on the light and looked into the powder room mirror. I saw the reflection of my face. I decided to begin my loving practice in the powder room mirror and so I announced to my reflection,

"I love you! I believe in the power of love. I am love."

CHAPTER FIFTEEN

Being Love

"You want me to write a book on self love?" I asked my face contorted in expressions that I could feel all the way to the back of my head. "Are you serious?"

"Yes," said Lori, my spiritual coach and advisor emphatically. "You are to write the quintessential book on self-love."

Lori, larger than life Lori, was not a person that I chose to mess with; she was powerful in spirit and in stature. And when she spoke, I always listened. However this announcement? This one was hard for me to believe. I was not sure what she was thinking. How could I write a book on self-love when I was as Idina Menzel sang in her song, "My Own Worst Enemy."[20]

I was harder on myself than I was with anyone else. And I realized that when I was hard on someone else, it was because I cared about him or her; I had convinced myself that the way that I love was to show up in a demanding way. I wasn't sure that was really all that loving. But I was sure that I showed up that way.

Lori interrupted my brooding mood and self-doubt with her confident empowering voice.

"I didn't hear you agree to this idea Marilee."

---

20   Idina Menzel, My Own Worst Enemy, from the album "I Stand".

Lori did not acknowledge my "hrumph" as a proper reply or dare I say, a valid reply. She asked me again.

"Marilee, do you doubt that you will be writing a book on how to become love; on how to be loving to yourself?"

"Doubt?" I exclaimed, sitting up in the chair that I had apparently slouched so far down into that it was as if I did a full gym-like sit up to get back upright and eye-to-eye with Lori who was sitting across the table from me.

"Doubt?" I repeated. "It is not doubt you are hearing in my voice; it is a declarative, are you fucking kidding me? I am so far out of the ability to love my self-category that I can't even imagine writing something like that. I think you have your clients confused Lori." With that obnoxious announcement left on the table, I slumped back into my chair, prepared to never sit up again.

Lori looked at me in silence for only a moment. I expected to hear some sort of pep talk from her, or some sort of direction on what I needed to do next. I wasn't looking at Lori; I was staring at my arms crossed in front of me, head, fully cocked forward, and shoulders hell bent forward in a dramatic sulking pose. I could feel Lori's eyes upon me however, so I looked up toward her direction. My eyes met hers and they locked. What I could see in Lori's gaze towards me was nothing short of love and an eerie kind of mystical wisdom. I shuddered. Lori waited for me to slowly slide upright again, roll my shoulders back, and then she spoke the final words of our visit.

"Just teach what you are learning Marilee. It will come to you." With that, she called for her assistant, who gathered up her papers from the table and they both melted into the background of the room.

I sat in the chair for a while, feeling the weight of my shoulders falling back toward my chest. I fought the urge to slump back into the chair and decided I would return to my usual humor that saved me from over-thinking so many times in the past. *I love that woman but I swear she makes shit up. I think she has me confused with someone else.* That thought gave me a smile and the energy I needed to push my shoulders back and rise, somewhat restored, from my chair for my long car drive back home.

The next day, I had a research meeting with one of my colleagues and I was frantically preparing last minute notes to discuss with the full research team. Another colleague peered into my office as I was gathering notes and re-writing key thoughts. I wanted to be ultra prepared for this meeting as the conference in which we were to present these results was fast approaching.

"Gotta minute?" I heard Alondra say as she peeked her head into my office.

What I wanted to say was, *if I had a minute, I would be spending it on trying to find the stinking analysis I mis-placed that we ran two weeks ago,* but something greater than me managed to keep my mouth closed. Instead, I spun around in my desk chair and surprised myself with the enthusiastic announcement of "Sure." I really was surprised at how energetic my response was; surely it was a nervous release from not being able to easily find the earlier data run.

Alondra stepped all the way into the office and shut the door. My immediate thought response and thankfully it stayed in my head and did not come out my mouth was, *you just shut the door. This is so going to take way longer than a minute.*

Alondra began to tell me her angst about having to fly up to Seattle that weekend to evict her brother and sister-in-law out of her flat. Apparently, she allowed them to live in her flat since she didn't want to sale it at the bottom of the market. However, they had failed to pay rent for three years. They were clearly taking advantage of her kindness.

"They haven't paid you anything in three years?" I exclaimed in disbelief.

"No," she said softly, tears welling up in her eyes. "I feel terrible doing this but I have asked and asked and they haven't even paid the $200/month that I asked them to a year ago as a good faith measure."

"$200/month?" I replied my mouth hanging open and my mind completely forgetting how much time had gone by since Alondra had closed the door to my office. "What does that place go for anyway?"

"Well," she paused. "Market value rent is about $2,800/month right now. It is a very nice place."

"Holy shit Alondra," I announced in my usual nonchalant way that always got a smile out of Alondra who is always so delicately proper and clearly amused by my crassness.

"Yes," she said the smile leaving her face. "I know, I know."

With that, I glanced down at my desk clock to note that my meeting time was fast approaching so I quickly explained to Alondra that our chat would have to be a short one. I sincerely apologized to her for this was a topic that deserved much more concentrated conversation. I knew that I would learn from this conversation, yet we were short on time. So, with the time that we had, I prayed for wisdom and shared what came with Alondra. I explained to Alondra that it seemed to me that she didn't love herself enough to ask her brother and sister-in-law to show up differently in this scenario. Alondra's face looked quizzically toward me and I surprised myself as I continued. I was not sure I was making sense but I was trusting the words as they came and so I shared them as they came.

I continued to explain to Alondra that as long as she was enabling her brother and sister-in-law to depend on her "good" nature to live in her place for free, she could feel that it was a surrogate for love. What I meant was that Alondra clearly didn't love herself enough to ask her brother and sister-in-law to pay her rent for her place. I reminded Alondra that her relatives were both working now and while they had been through tough times, so had Alondra. However, Alondra was confusing the co-dependent situation – the seeming kindness of allowing her family to live in her place rent-free – for love. What it really was, was a bad replacement for love. Alondra was keeping her family in need of her instead of allowing them to stand on their own and allowing authentic love to blossom. How could love be expressed in a situation where Alondra had created an opportunity for her family to simply become dependent on her? Alondra said that she resented her family taking advantage of her but it seemed more to me that she was afraid to ask them to pay the rent for fear that she would lose their dependence on her and in so doing, she would lose her surrogate for love.

"That ain't self-love Alondra. That's akin to paying someone to date you." As I finished my monologue, I noticed Alondra's face. All the color had left it. I asked her if I had said too much. Alondra declared that she was OK, but I felt that she really wasn't.

"Look Alondra, I am not saying that you are doing this to be evil. I am saying that it appears to me that you haven't thought about whether your so called generosity is really love motivated or whether it is motivated by fear of losing the presence of your brother and sister-in-law in your life. It seems to me that you are afraid to demand that they pay rent because they have become so dependent on you and you like that dependence. You don't want to lose that because it keeps them in your life and you may think that is love. Well Alondra, I know I am no expert, but seriously, that is like the time I kept allowing this guy I was dating to eat all my food. Remember Alex? He lost his job and I felt for him and I thought it would be loving to let him have a key to my place so he could eat while he was trying to get back on his feet. But then he kept coming over a lot and eating a lot and it was costing me a lot. But yet, I really loved the time with him. I was afraid that if I told him to stop, he would quit hanging around and I really liked him hanging around. But the truth was, I couldn't' afford him eating me out of house and home. Finally, I decided that I wasn't being loving to him or to me. I wasn't helping him get back on his feet by allowing this to happen, all I was doing was enabling him to become dependent on me and I was paying a huge price for his attention. That ain't love sister."

Alondra sat in silence and nodded her head. I saw the clock ticking but I wanted to make one more point about what this conversation was teaching me.

"Alondra, what I am learning is that every time I become resentful about something I think I am doing in love, I realize that what is at the heart of it is the simple truth that I don't love myself enough to show up authentically and say what I really feel or what I really mean. There is no doubt in my mind that you love your brother and his wife and that you allowed them to stay at your place rent free to help them out. But now, three years later, when they are working again, you are still allowing it. Why is that?"

Tears began to stream down Alondra's face. I moved over to the chair where she was sitting and gave her a tight hug. I handed her my box of Kleenex but she didn't try to pull tissues from it. She just sat, head drooped, motionless in my chair.

"Sweetie, you are worthy of love. I recognized that when I realized that Alex was eating me out of house and home and I was growing resentful, I had moved out of providing for him from a place of genuine love to providing for him out of a place where I didn't trust that I was worth hanging out with unless I fed him. It was a crazy idea – the idea that I had to keep feeding this man in order for him to feel as if I was worthy to hang around. Well, I am worthy. And Alondra, so are you."

Her streaming tears became a waterfall and I found myself grabbing the tissues from the box to hand her but she still didn't respond. I found myself feeling a little anxious now. For one, it was well past the time that my meeting was to have started. Secondly, and of course more importantly, I had someone that I loved dearly in my office crying and I had no idea what to do next. So, I held onto Alondra with all my strength and prayed for clarity.

A soft tap on my office door came next. The sound of it startled both Alondra and me and we jumped slightly which made us giggle. It was a welcome release for both of us. I called to the person behind the door that I would be there in a moment. The tender voice that simply said,

"OK" was a voice I recognized as one of my colleagues with whom I was to meet.

Alondra and I decided that the best thing to do was for her to sit and rest in my office while I stole away to attend my meeting. We both promised each other we would check in with each other later. I grabbed my research papers hurriedly and sloppily and made my way out the door of my office careful not to open the door too widely in an attempt not to reveal Alondra's presence still within my office. But this maneuver required more grace than I had and the papers I was holding fell to the ground scattering everywhere. I managed to close my door, realizing I had left both my keys and laptop in the office but at this point, I really didn't care.

Lonni, the colleague who had tapped so lightly on the door prior was right there to help me pick up the scattered papers. We were both kneeling on the floor grabbing what we could as quickly as we could. As I looked up to thank her, I noticed that her eyes were red. Their appearance startled me. The end of semesters were hard on everyone but Lonni's eyes looked as if she was either getting sick with something or worse…in mourning.

"Lonni? Why are your eyes red?" Well that was either the best question I could ask or the worst. Lonni's eyes glistened and she explained to me that she was not fully prepared for our meeting. She was apologizing profusely and was going on and on with explanations of why she was not prepared when I finally sat back onto the floor with my bum hitting the carpet hard.

"Ouch!" I yelled so loudly that it disrupted Lonni's trance-like monologue and she seemed to be shaken back to reality and surprised that I was seated on the floor directly in front of her. I think she honestly had forgotten that I was there. "Sorry Lonni." I said half giggling. "I lost my balance."

"It is OK," Lonni said with relatively no emotion and returned to what seemed her highest duty in picking up and organizing the papers I had dropped.

"Uh Lonni," my hand reached to grab her arm. I intended to hold her arm and shake her back to the plane where I was residing. She seemed to be completely absent.

"Lonni," I said again this time making the physical connection that I had intended to occur. "Lonni," I repeated now trying to get her eyes to connect with mine. "What's going on? What happened?"

"Lonni's eyes would not meet mine and I knew something was terribly wrong. I grabbed the remaining papers, lifted Lonni up with my free arm and guided her to the meeting room where our research meeting was to take place. We were the only ones there. Apparently, the rest of my colleagues had given up on us. I would address that later. It was just going to have to wait. In this moment, the research had been forgotten. Clearly, the Universe had other plans for my day.

With my free hand, I closed the door behind us, placed the stack of crumpled papers on the meeting table, and pulled out a chair for Lonni to sit. My other hand was still holding Lonni's arm guiding her as gently as I was able to into the chair.

I asked Lonni again what was happening and she proceeded to explain. I knew that Lonni's mom, Sarah, was having a terrible battle with cancer and I knew that Sarah depended on Lonni to be her primary caregiver, her chauffer, and her primary source of strength. I had watched Lonni in great admiration as she handled this pressure with loving care amidst the other duties and responsibilities she shouldered. I was in awe at how well she was managing it all. And in this moment, I was still in respectful awe at her although I was feeling more of deep concern for what could possibly be causing her this much pain and anguish and the "out-of-body" type existence. I felt my body shiver as Lonni reminded me of what I already knew about the extent of care she was providing her mom.

Lonni continued and she shared how she had become frustrated with her mom for depending so much on her for the care-giving. Lonni wanted her mom to ask her father for assistance and also to ask her brother for assistance, especially since he had recently flown into help out with the care-giving. I encouraged Lonni by congratulating her for asking for help – something that we all struggled with doing and I told Lonni how I respected her for asking for what she needed. Lonni's response startled me.

"Yeah, sure Marilee. I asked and then my mom got angry at me and now I am feeling incredibly guilty." Lonni spoke with the tone of a five-year-old who was telling a friend that the advice they had been given basically sucked and had gotten them into more trouble. And so, I couldn't help but burst into laughter. I had been so worried that something else had happened. This? This was not what I expected to hear. And clearly my response was not what Lonni had expected either.

"Why are you laughing at me Marilee? This isn't funny."

"I am so sorry Lonni; you are right. It isn't funny at all. I am sorry. It is just the way you said it that made it sound like you were five-years-old and…" I stopped short of my explanation as Lonni's scowl caught my eyes.

"I am sorry Lonni." I repeated and Lonni continued without seemingly taking a breath.

"I feel guilty for telling my mom that I just couldn't help her today. After all, my brother is here and my dad took off a day of work. They can take her to her chemo treatment and god knows I need a break from all of this. I am exhausted."

I encouraged Lonni to continue and she looked at me rather inquisitively as if to suggest I might burst into laughter again. However, the laughter had long since passed. I was not sure why Lonni was feeling guilty for requesting a much-needed break. I was more interested in learning about that than in learning what Lonni had told her mom in order to convince her mom that her dad and brother could take care of her as well as she could. Lonni seemed convinced that my urging for her to continue to share was sincere. After only a slight hesitation, she continued with her story.

Lonni shared that even though she knew that she was tired and needed a break that she found that she was feeing guilty about asking for a break from tending to her mom. I shared back that I understood this to be "normal"; that often caregivers feel exhausted by the care they are providing but don't feel that they can or should take a break. However, in this case, it was clear that she wasn't abandoning her mother for her mother had her husband, Lonni's dad, and her son, Lonni's brother, to care for her. In addition, there were several friends who would also be happy to give Lonni a break but Lonni's mother didn't want them to see her in the state she was currently in – having no hair and feeling sick and weak. Yet, Lonni's mom lived with her husband so that one… that one I didn't understand.

Lonni continued to explain that she had made this research meeting appointment with just me and not the entire team. She had also made reservations at one of our favorite beach restaurants for this time. Her plan had been to pick me up and take me there as a surprise; she knew I wouldn't leave work unless it was for work. It was finally dawning on me that I didn't need to prepare anything for this meeting for it really wasn't a research meeting at all and that also helped explain where everyone else was; they weren't coming. I hadn't even missed them. I was the only one who knew about the alleged meeting that was really suppose to be a lunch on the beach between two friends – one who desperately needed a light hearted break from her mother's circumstances.

Upon hearing that we had luncheon reservations at George's bistro with the amazing view of the ocean, I didn't want to waste one more minute in the cramped window-less conference room that we were occupying. I pulled Lonni out of her chair, almost pulling her arm out of her socket, dropped my research papers off at the reception desk for fear I that I would disturb Alondra who might still be sitting in my office, yelled something like "we are taking our meeting off campus so you can free up the conference room" and almost ran out of the office building still with Lonni in tow. As we slid into Lonni's car, I asked her again. I just wanted to make sure I wasn't skipping out on something I was suppose to be attending.

"So, we don't have a research team meeting?"

"No," Lonni said a little sheepishly as she pulled onto the somewhat crowded interstate. It was Friday and the traffic to the beach was always busy on Friday afternoons.

"I knew that if I told you I needed a break, you wouldn't take a break from work. I knew I had to pitch it as a work meeting in order to get you out of the office to join me for a lunch outing."

I laughed aloud at first letting Lonni know that she was exactly right and then I realized that what she had said really wasn't funny at all. One of my best friends desperately needed a break during the middle of the day and she knew I wouldn't take a break from my work unless she scheduled a work meeting. I felt disappointed; I wasn't disappointed by Lonni's actions, I was disappointed that what she said about me was true.

"And what did you tell your folks?" I asked, wondering if she told them she was going to work as well.

"The same thing." Her face grimaced. "I told them I had to go to work. I had to have this meeting. It was important."

We both sat in silence with the weight of what we both felt we had to say and do in order to simply go have an extended lunch on a workday at one of our most favorite places to eat.

"Is that bad?" Lonni inquired. "Is what I did wrong?" I could hear her voice beginning to quiver.

"Well," I said. "Before you start feeling guilty about anything else, remember that we are in this one together. I knew full well I wasn't headed to a meeting when I practically ran out the door and announced that I *was* headed to a meeting to the entire working world."

Lonni giggled and I was grateful to hear her mood lighten. She spoke a while longer recapping the entire discussion she had had with her mom, her dad, and her brother. She had spent a lot of energy to have these moments away from caring for her mom and it seemed to me that so far, the investment had not been worth it to her. She was still weighed down. However, this time, she was not weighed down by the burden of care-giving, she was weighed down by the way she had removed herself from the situation.

"Lonni," I interrupted her as she began to repeat the entire scenario and detailed conversation for the third time. "Let's break this down piece-by-piece, shall we?" She paused a moment from her story and then simply nodded in agreement.

"So, are you authentically and genuinely pleased that you made the decision to not take your mom back and forth from her chemo treatment today?"

"Yes, but...I feel guilty about not being there for her."

I rudely and abruptly interrupted Lonni. I didn't want to hear the same story again. So I repeated the question and asked that she provide a simple yes or no answer with no buts.

"Lonni, are you authentically and genuinely pleased that you made the decision to not take your mom back and forth from her chemo treatment today?"

"Yes," she said and the grimace returned to her face.

"Well, I am authentically very happy to be here with you on this glorious day on our way to the beach for lunch at one of our favorite restaurants." I announced loudly. The declaration brought a smile to Lonni's face replacing the pain-filled grimace for a moment and then the grimace retuned.

"But I feel guilty about it all." She said again.

Taking a deep sigh, I asked her to clarify whether she felt guilty about the choice or the way in which she communicated her choice to her family? Lonni remained silent in response. I could tell she was doing a great deal of thinking. So I decided to share what I was feeling.

"Lonni, I am so happy to be going to lunch with you. Just a moment ago, however, I had pangs of guilt for going to lunch with you."

Lonni's grimace worsened in its expression.

"Let me explain Lonni." I continued. "First, I felt guilty for lying to everyone at work about what I am doing. I am going to lunch with you – not having a research meeting. Why did I lie and say we were meeting off-site? I didn't lie because I think there is anyone at work who would shame me for going to lunch; they wouldn't. I lied because I don't think I deserve to have a lunch break when I am so behind on so many things. Then again, maybe I don't think I deserve a lunch break period. Whatever the reason, I choose right now to let all that shit go. I am thrilled to be going to lunch with you and I am not going to allow this voice in my head that says I should be working instead to get in the way of this choice. Does that make sense?"

Lonni nodded and I could tell she was thinking more about what we were discussing than the road upon which she was driving but I wasn't worried about our safety whatsoever.

"Lonni, do you think you can let go of your guilt long enough to enjoy the very reason that you made this luncheon reservation in the first place? Do you think you can just try on believing that you deserve this break so that you can fully enjoy it?"

Lonni nodded again and I saw a smile make its way slowly onto her face. I was delighted. We drove on further and I shifted the conversation to lighter topics. Lonni eased into the conversation and I did as well. We were catching each other up on the guys that we were each dating, the summer clothes we wanted to purchase but knew we wouldn't and the dream vacations we would like to take with our current boyfriends. We even played around with double dating ideas. Before we knew it, we had both forgotten that we were supposed to be doing other things and enjoying the moment with each other, the gorgeous view, and the delightful food. We even ordered a glass of wine; something I never let myself do during the middle of a work-day.

As we strolled along the beachfront ensuring our wine had worn off completely before getting back into the car for our drive back to my workplace, we returned to our earlier conversation. We spoke at length about our inability to authentically express what we need. We gave each other several examples of how we do what we think we should do instead of really owning that which we do do or want to do. We decided that it came down to our inability to publicly display our love of ourselves. We have an aversion to self-PDA (public display of affection). We laughed so hard at this idea but then once again, we realized that it wasn't really funny. We drove on in silence.

"Why do you think we don't love ourselves enough to tell the world we are going to go to the beach for a lunch in the middle of a work day?" I asked interrupting our thoughts with a question that I did not intend to be hypothetical. "It is not like we will ever make a habit out of this? Or will we?" I giggled about the idea of doing this every day but I was all by myself in my expression of humor. Lonni was in silence, so I answered my own question.

"Lonni, you and I get to embark on a journey now where we get to challenge ourselves and each other to genuinely ask for what we authentically need. No more performing as the people that others expect for us to be. If you get tired of caring for your mom, you tell someone that you need help and you are not to worry about whether you will look like a bad daughter. Deal?" I said, extending my hand over to one of her hands that was grasping the car wheel as if to shake on this concept.

Lonni glanced over toward me with a grin on her face. Extending her hand towards mine she agreed and offered me a challenge to consider as well.

"And you Marilee, you will allow yourself to have a social lunch in the middle of the work day and tell people you are having a social lunch in the middle of the work day regardless of whether they will think you are a slacker for doing so. Deal?"

Laughing I shook her hand enthusiastically and yelled "deal" loud enough to frighten the folks passing us by in their cars. We giggled a bit more and then spoke once more of ideal double dates that we could take our boyfriends on together. We chatted about nothing at all until we got closer to my work. As we drew near my workplace, I could feel my anxiety rise. I realized I had just been on a 3-hour lunch and I had so much work to do before boarding the plan the next day to head to a conference. My head was filled with wrestling thoughts wondering if I would be able to keep to the deal that I had made less than an hour prior.

Thanking Lonni for her brilliant "meeting" idea and for the very helpful conversation, I slid out of her car and walked toward my office. I knew it would be a late night of work for me. I knew I would be "making up the hours" that I had spent at lunch and I wasn't sure if that had to do with my lack of self-love or simply my responsibility to my job and to my constituents.

I guess what really matters in all of this is when I need a break, when I truly need a break, will I genuinely show up in authenticity and ask for it or will I feign an excuse or tell a lie? Will I worry more about what others think of me because I asked for a break? Or will I be able to be authentic and just say, hey I need a fucking break here. I am going to lunch. I intend to state that I need a break —without inserting the word fucking — and then take it. Wow! How refreshing will that be to everyone — eh? I like this authenticity stuff. Authenticity and self-love. They go together very nicely, don't they?

CHAPTER SIXTEEN

Being In-Love

"What does it mean to me to be in love?" Larger than life Lori asked me this; it was the last question of our coaching session together. I didn't know. So as I left my life coaching appointment with her, once again, she gave me an assignment. She asked me to journal about this question. She asked me to quit gathering data on what everyone else thought this answer was for them and simply write about it from my heart; what would my heart say if a posed this question to that space.

And so I did journal about it, but not until I was crossing on the ferry from Vancouver Island to Vancouver city, nine days after I met the man who would inspire me to dig so deeply within and consider whether I was ready to answer this question.

What does it mean for me to be in love? I don't know.

Traveling on the ferry from Vancouver Island to Vancouver city, transitioning from a 2-day retreat to full on work mode, it just struck me (*I love it when that happens*) that it was time to answer this question. So, after I parked my rented very red, very used Kia automobile on deck number four of this massive ferry, I grabbed my laptop and headed up to the passenger deck to find a space, gaze at the incredible view, and be inspired. The breath-taking scenery was indeed inspiring, as was the people watching – several hundreds running all around me, chatting in a number of languages and engaged in all sorts of activities from playing cards to sleeping to enjoying the natural beauty that I was enjoying to talking about genomics (yes, genomics). But even more inspirational were the prior email and phone conversations I was having with the man I had met only 9 days prior. His name was Ruben. All of this contributed to my journal writing in the moment.

I watch couples around me who appear to be in love and those who appear to be in comfortable relationships that are...well...just comfortable. I mean they appear to be content with one another but not really attentive to each other. So, I guess, I would expect that to be what "in love" means. To be "in love" means that I would be attentive to my partner's needs and expressions, as I would expect he would be attentive to mine. I would be more than just comfortable and resting, I would be actively engaged with him and in that engagement, I would find respite and peace.

Yet, I would not expect him to be more attentive to me than he is to himself. What I mean by that is that it would be hard for me to know what he needs if he isn't aware enough of his own needs to know them first. Thus, I wouldn't want to be so lost in attending to my partners' needs and desires that I would not know mine first. In this sense, we would each be responsible for knowing our own selves first and thus, it would allow us to fully tend to each other. This would allow us to practice authentic self-love so as to fully express and feel the self-in-love.

So, to be in love means that I can't wait to see him again once I part his side. Of course, we would be apart daily, for the coming together again would be joyous. If we never parted, we wouldn't know the joy and ecstasy of joining once again. Yet, to be in love means that I wouldn't want to be apart from him for long periods of time for my yearning for his presence would be a longing that I wouldn't want to prolong. It would simply be too painful - the yearning for him would ring to loudly with an echo of emptiness, a void. Apart from him, my soul would become restless to find her mate and in so doing the resonance of its anxiety to re-connect would send waves of chaos all around me. My aching heart would disrupt the peace that typically encompasses me and all of nature around me would feel its disruption.

No, it would not be wise for the Universe to have me be apart from my Love for too long.

To be in love means an over riding sense of compassion and joy and tenderness between he and me. In every word and in every gesture, all one can see is pure unabashed love and peace, joy and tenderness, and respect and admiration. Yet, when we are alone and in a space where we can join as one physically, the unbridled union resonates within every cell of my being and within his. The shrieks of ecstasy replace the tender words spoken in public and the animal-like desire for closeness means my skin becomes one with his as do our lips, eyes, heart, and soul. Our union re-defines metaphysical explanations and the transparency of our Oneness astounds all those who see us together. They describe us as mystical and we laugh upon hearing this. We know it is not mystical, rather it just is as it was designed to be. And we express our gratitude for having the opportunity to experience this Oneness within these bodies and within this life.

To be in love means that when we are apart, we feel each other's presence and support and coaching. We are uplifted to be our best for our individual selves and for our united selves. We selflessly give from our abundance storehouse of love to those around us. And this storehouse is easily replenished when we gaze upon each other uniting again within each other's arms, legs entwined, hearts merged, and souls afire.

To be in love is to experience time suspended, to know that its passing is an illusion and to feel the truth of our togetherness as untouchable by disease, knowledge, judgment, or death of our bodies. To be in love is to experience for the first time the Universal truth that we are all connected and to feel everything, every thought, every encounter, every word spoken or song heard so deeply that we are moved always beyond the words we have been given to express how we feel.

To be in love, to truly be in love, is the greatest gift of all gifts, the greatest adventure of all life times, and the greatest peace that could ever be known. There are no fears to be experienced when one is in love; there are no losses to be felt. There is only the joy and exhilaration of the experience.

To be in love is to live a life more fully, freely, and generously than one ever could imagine living it before. To be in love is to know God, to experience God, and to be One with God in every moment and in every way.

I invite this sense of being into my life. I welcome it and I embrace it. And for once in my life, it is possible for me to even imagine it. Thank you mountains and sea for your beauty. Thank you Ruben for your inspiration! Thank you Lori for this assignment! Thank you God for allowing this to be love! This is something to which I am delighted to surrender.

CHAPTER SEVENTEEN

Invitation Only

"Ya know? I am going to have to disagree with you on that one." I said rather emphatically to Bob. Bob, an avid ACIM and Tao practitioner, taught me a great deal about many things. He was always generously sharing his wisdom, readings, and sending me citations from all sorts of publications for my use in my teaching and my own daily spiritual practice. If it wasn't for Bob, I would not have been introduced to so many different spiritual teachers, teachings, practices, and perspectives. I was truly grateful for Bob. However, in this moment and on this particular topic, I didn't care how many citations he had, I was done listening.

"Well here is another source of this same teaching Marilee. This one is from Colin Tipping. [21]He states clearly here that you invite in all the lessons from which you need to learn. Thus Marilee, you have invited this particular situation into your life, so what is it that you need to learn from this?"

Bob, as Bob so often did, was getting excited about the conversation now. It seemed that when it came to my conversations with Bob, the more I wanted to end the conversation, the more he became engaged. Furthermore, the particular situation to which he was referring was a

---

21   Radical Forgiveness Steps from Colin Tipping – http://www.
     radicalforgiveness.com/

painful one. He was referring to his perspective that it was a fact that I had invited into my life the intruder that placed a tub of black clothing underneath my bed. The tub that contained a black full-face ski mask, turtleneck, gloves, and pants; the clothing that to me represented intent to either rob my neighbors or rape me. Bob was explaining to me that I had invited that experience into my life because there was a lesson that I needed to learn from that experience.

"Ya know Bob… seriously… we need to end this conversation. We are moving from a loving conversation to one that looks more like a debate. You want to convince me that the perspective you are teaching me is the right one and I want to hold onto the perspective that I now have. So, please let it go for now. I am done listening and when I am done listening, I can no longer learn."

The tone in my voice had moved to the tone I use in the classroom when I am giving one of my very opinionated lectures. I was praying that Bob was not only hearing my tone change; I was praying that he was also really listening to my words. I was being authentic here; when I latch onto an idea or perspective, I no longer listen. And when I no longer listen, I no longer learn.

After a few more back and forth comments, Bob took the cues that were increasing in dynamics and let the conversation go. When he let the conversation go, I took the opportunity to also physically leave his presence. I so appreciated all that Bob taught me but I often left conversations with him feeling drained. I know he didn't intend to and I know he just got excited about what he was teaching, but I always felt like he was trying to convince me to adopt his perspective rather than approach the conversation from inquiry and exploration. I left conversations with Bob feeling judged, rather than feeling free to explore. According to Bob and ACIM, that was all of my own doing. And obviously, there was a lesson for me to learn there. I just didn't know what it was in this moment. Furthermore, I did not appreciate the lesson he was teaching me in this moment.

In this moment, the teaching that we invite everything, absolutely everything, into our lives so that we can learn the lesson it has to teach us aggravated me. According to Bob's explanation of ACIM and according to Colin Tipping, I had asked for this black tub of clothing to be placed under my bed by some intruder, similarly to their interpretation that I had asked to be raped because there was a lesson there for me to learn. In addition, this meant that one of my best friend's mother had cancer because she had asked for it and another one of my friend's twin son's died because she had invited that in as well. So, you get the picture... way too much for my brain to handle in this moment.

I was basically annoyed and I was convinced that the folks who taught this stuff and really believed it never had been raped, survived cancer, or lost a child. They must have learned their lessons from observing others or reading about it in books and didn't need the life experiences that the rest of us needed in order to learn what they already knew. So, what I decided I needed in this moment, was a long hike on Cowle's mountain. I needed to let go of the pain that this teaching was causing me. I needed to let go of the self-judgment that I was apparently a masochistic dunce given all the experiences I had invited into my life. I needed to let go of trying to figure this shit out.

Hiking on Cowles Mountain, or Meditation Mountain, which I had come to lovingly call it, was always a pleasant respite. I loved how release always came from walking on this sacred mountain and sometimes, clarity even came with the release. As I began the hike up the mountain following my bow and request for permission to walk its path, two men quickly passed me by. They were power walking, something I never attempted on the mountain. They power walked by me so quickly, all I heard from their conversation and I wasn't even trying to listen to them was,

"And then all of a sudden she changed. And I discovered I was dating someone I didn't even know."

The comment caused me to stop in my path. My first thought was *I wondered what lesson he needed to learn that caused him to invite that situation into his life.* I found myself trying to think of some response that would make me laugh so as to get back out of my head, but nothing came, so I continued to walk on.

Directly in front of me, hiking down the mountain was another pair of men. They were also walking quickly and as if a message were being given to me through them, I heard another phrase, oddly similar to the first one.

"I don't know. It was just like she had become a completely different person…"

I found myself stopping once again in my tracks. This is weird. I glanced back to the beginning of the path. I hadn't even walked 100 yards and I had heard two separate pairs of men basically speaking about the same topic. I understood them to be concerned with the women they were dating. Apparently the women suddenly and unexpectedly changed.

I giggled to myself and realized that I don't think they invited any of that into their lives. No doubt these were women who were trying to be something they weren't in order to get these men to like being with them and either the women decided a) these guys were not worth keeping the show up for or they simply b) just got tired of their made-up lives and decided it was time to become real. I would have to tell Bob that this was an example of something that I didn't think these men invited into their lives for them to learn a lesson – it was a result of a couple of women most likely being inauthentic and then deciding to be authentic or vice versa. Who knew?

I walked along a little longer realizing I was not going to be able to shake Bob's lesson from my mind. What I knew I did believe was that discoveries *can* occur from everyday life happenings and from traumatic life experiences. The lessons I had learned from being raped, from losing the use of my legs, from losing loved ones, and even from losing a pair of earrings were all quite profound and there was no doubt in my mind that I felt I had grown into a more loving person from each and every one of these instances. But to think that I had invited them into my life; *why the fuck would I do that?*

I walked along in silence, now completely unaware of who may be passing by me. I was lost in my thoughts.

I believe I am god and that everyone I see on this path is also god. I believe that we are all connected and that we are all One. I do not wish for any one of god's creatures to experience pain or suffering nor do I wish that I experience any of it. I recognize that my ego may have made me a more stubborn student of life and I acknowledge that many of my lessons have had to be learned the hard way, however, my new way of being is of love and of light and still, I encounter anger and violence within my life. Am I inviting these experiences in so that I can practice being love and light? Or are these things just happening because as the physicists say, opposites attract and like repels[22]? But even in the physics analogy for opposites to attract or like to repel, something must be positively charged while something else is simply neutral. Could it be that all of these events are neither good nor bad, rather, they just are life experiences? And could it be that it is within me to either make them into positive learnings or horrible messes?

Even though my mind was in a whirlwind of chatter, I did notice the large colorful lizard that crossed my path, so I stepped to the side of the path to watch it walk nonchalantly into the bushes in front of me. My thoughts and my walking seized while I admired this magnificent creature making its way without a seeming care in the world from bush to bush. The lizard was the creature known by the Shamans as being able to detach its tail from its body when its life was threatened only to grow one anew. As I understood from the Shaman teachings[23], the tail of the Lizard was equated to the ego of man. The lizard could detach its tail − its ego − very quickly when the tail - the ego − caused the lizard's life to be threatened. The story of the lizard's tale and its parable of the human ego had caused me to become more aware of my own choices and my own mindfulness of my ability or inability to detach myself from my ego should it be threatening my spiritual or physical well-being in any way.

Was I now needing to detach the tail of my ego in order to accept Bob's lesson as truth? Or was there something else I was to be learning here from all of this chaos that had recently found its way into my home?

My mind returned to the comments that I had overheard from the two pairs of men walking the same path upon which I walked; the comments that seemed to allude to women suddenly changing in their

---

22   http://www.physicsclassroom.com/class/estatics/u8l1e.cfm
23   http://www.animalspirits.com/index.html

lives, suddenly becoming people they no longer knew or thought they knew. I recognized there could be several reasons for these men to have experienced this, however in this moment a very specific thought struck me.

Maybe it is our individual in-authenticity that leads us to life's experiences that required us to learn tough lessons? But wait, how would that apply to the examples I had given Bob earlier? How would this, for instance, apply to my being raped.

The lesson I chose to take away from my rape was to trust my inner voice; the voice that screams out, *you better not walk down this road and into this building. You better just take a cab. Quit trying to save money when your well-being is at stake.*

And what I learned from that lesson – that very tough lesson is to trust my inner voice. The voice that says, *this is what you need to do in this situation right now, so do it* instead of minimizing the inner voice with an often over-riding voice that comes from a sense of a lack of self-love or a concern for not offending anyone or a concern for looking good.

I did not accept the teaching that so many people tell someone that has had this experience. Stupid messages get sent like, you should have known better than to walk from the train to your hotel by yourself, you should have known better than to be nice to that man who offered to escort you from the train station to your hotel room. You should have, you should have, you should have…

The only *should have* in the situation that led to my rape was that I didn't listen to my inner voice and I *should have* listened to it. I had traveled to foreign countries by myself many times. I had taken the kind gestures of men and women to escort me from one place to another and each time in those instances, my inner voice had said, *no worries. This is cool.* I didn't have some inauthentic rule that didn't apply to my soul. In the situations where no harm was done and only good occurred, I listened to my inner truth. When I didn't listen to my inner truth, when I was concerned about hurting someone else's feelings, someone I had just meant, and when I was concerned about saving money more than tending to my own well-being, I got raped. Did I invite that lesson into my life? Or was a situation presented to me and I chose to learn from it? It certainly feels better to me to choose the latter belief.

I don't believe that my dear friend invited in the loss of one of her twin sons because she needed to learn the lesson that could only be learned from that situation. I don't believe my friends who have cancer invited cancer in so they could learn what needed to be learned from that. I don't believe that when my cousin was blown to bits in Beirut that he invited that into his life – he didn't live to learn whatever fucking lesson he was to learn from that. So what does that mean; that I invited him to be blown to bits because I told him that there were other ways to experience adventure and serve your country than joining the Marines? No, I don't believe we invite shit into our lives. I do believe however, that we can accept the crap that has come into our life as "crap that just happened to come into our life." I believe that we can learn from whatever experiencing that "crap" will teach us, if we choose to learn from it and remain open to whatever growth in love comes from experiencing it. And I do believe, that we can choose not to fabricate an intricate story around the stuff that happens. Just choose to see it as stuff that happens, nothing more.

I believe the same is true for all the joys that come into our lives. I am so richly blessed. I don't believe that all the blessings have come into my life because I invited them in. I believe that I am open to experiencing them and learning from them as much as I am open to experiencing the crap of life and learning from it as well.

Maybe that is just it, I am simply an energetic conduit – perhaps a positively charged proton interacting with neutral experiences, translating to the best of my ability all that happens to me, making meaning of it, learning from it, and sharing what I learned with others. It ain't voo doo, it is just physics, pure and simple.

All of my life experiences have taught me many lessons, some of which are what you would expect, such as discovering how precious life is, what a gift it is to breathe, to see, to hear, to walk, to talk, to laugh, to sing, and to dance. I have been given the privilege to discover that every moment is a gift and that peace comes from choosing acceptance and love, joy comes from being present in each and every moment, even when you are experiencing emotional or physical pain beyond what you believe you can bear. For it is as the wise men say, "this too shall pass[24]," even when the passing feels like it will take for-fucking-ever.

I believe that choosing anger and resentment can provide immediate comfort; but in time, it only fuels more anger and resentment, which then fuels fear and that leads to in-authenticity. And in fear, I find no joy or peace and fewer opportunities to choose Love. I believe that God, the Creator, the Universe - I actually have no idea what to name "it" - but "it" is that which is Source Power and that which resides within each one of us gives me the strength to, in time, choose Love. When I forget to choose love, it is because I have experienced a great misunderstanding of who I am and who you are. The Source Power resides in you and in me. You are god and I am god. I am often reminded of who I am because of you and all the lessons you teach me. And all these lessons, invited or not, reaffirm my commitment to being or becoming my authentic self - to becoming Love.

---

24   http://www.wscribe.com/parables/pass.html

CHAPTER EIGHTEEN

Being Greatness

"I just realized that we spend our entire lives trying to down play our uniqueness – our own authenticity - trying to fit into an expectation that others have of us or that society has of us – whatever... Basically, we spend a lifetime trying to hide our greatness, our beauty, our brilliance. No wonder it takes us so damn long to become authentic again. Since we first learn to utter words and walk, we get socialized to "fit in", to become invisible, to not draw attention to ourselves. And even those who end up drawing attention to themselves are not doing so out of their greatness, they are doing so out of their lack of love for themselves. They are doing so out of their lack of authenticity. So what does it mean to be authentic? What does it mean to step into our greatness?"

"Whoa Kelsey!" I exclaimed as I looked into her eyes as she finished her rant. "What just happened?"

I had just met Kelsey for a quick cup of tea at the end of the day, or should I say at the end of most people's workday (5:00 p.m.), but which was typically just half way in between ours since we often used the evening to write or to grade papers when we weren't teaching at night.

Kelsey let out what sounded like the mix between a moan and a grunt and a slight growl, as she began to explain to me that she had just come out of her consultation for her re-appointment to teach another year. She was frustrated about what she had heard. She felt like she had been given a mixture of congratulations on the result of her creative expression and a bit of what also sounded a lot like "get back in the box" that you keep crawling out of while demonstrating all your creativity.

I listened to the frustration in her voice and saw the pain in her eyes. She was experiencing something I knew all too well and hadn't been successful at maneuvering either – the challenge of finding your own voice while knowing you still have to play "by the rules" to get the creative voice heard.

"I am sick of it Marilee. I am sick of it. How am I suppose to step into my authenticity and maintain it while I am being told that if I don't do this and that, I will lose the very venue that allowed me to explore my creativity in the first place?"

I could see that Kelsey's painful eyes were trying to determine whether they would begin to flash in anger or break into tears of sorrow. I wanted to say something helpful but all that came out was,

"That's a damn good question Kelsey. I have no idea."

I really felt at a loss for words but apparently, my honesty in having no idea how to respond to Kelsey and not even being able to be creative enough to make up some sort of response or make her laugh was enough to remove some of the pain in her eyes. Kelsey began to smile as she chided me playfully for not being very helpful at all. It was a nice feeling, for once in my life, to have a state of not knowing bring a smile to someone else's face.

"Seriously Marilee, how do you do it? How do you be authentic and keep people off your back so you can remain authentic?"

Now I was the one laughing and I was laughing so loudly that the baristas who prepare our favorite foo foo coffee and tea beverages were wondering what joke they had missed and were inviting Kelsey to re-tell it. Kelsey glanced at them impatiently for having interrupted our conversation, explained briefly to them that there was no joke, that I had just lost my mind momentarily again.

The baristas were accustomed to my loud outbursts of laughter so they inquired no more and returned to their work. All seemed back to normal behind the coffee service counter, even though I continued to laugh aloud.

"Kelsey, you know I practice what I am learning and I share what I need to learn. I don't do anything well and I have no answers." I spoke still giggling but trying to calm my laughter as I had my very favorite green tea soy latte, no classic, no foam in my hand. I was excited about taking my first sip.

"OK, OK," Kelsey said with her impatience growing by the moment. "Tell me what you are learning then. Tell me about what you are practicing. What do you think authenticity is and how do you 'do' it in light of everyone around you asking you to simply play games?"

"Damn good questions" I repeated but this time neither of us thought I was funny. I told Kelsey about how I had just gone to yoga class[25] that morning where the instructor defined what authenticity was. She spoke to us as we began our integration series of yoga and she told us that being authentic was the willingness to be with what we felt and thought and to be OK with those feelings and thoughts. As I listened to her speak about being authentic, I thought of the irony of my having looked this word up in the on-line Merriam Webster dictionary just two days prior. In the dictionary, I had read that authentic had been defined as "true to one's own personality, spirit, or character."[26] It was interesting to me how the yoga instructor's explanation landed more solidly on me than did the dictionary definition.

I explained to Kelsey that I understood authenticity to be just what my yoga instructor said that it was. That in simply acknowledging that when I was angry, I was angry and that was my authentic self. To be angry and then tell my self why I shouldn't be angry was not authentic. Yes, there would be a time for acknowledging the anger and then exploring it, but that was part of the authentic process. Feeling angry

---

25   Core Power Yoga, San Diego, CA
26   Merriam-Webster on-line dictionary; http://www.merriam-webster.com/dictionary/authentic

and pretending not to be angry because someone thinks I shouldn't be that way was not authentic.

I could see Kelsey's furrowed brow as I spoke so I shared a few more examples.

"You know, it is like when I am in a meeting and someone starts speaking about something I don't care about and I think, 'I don't care about this at all. I am not even interested in this topic and furthermore, I don't agree with the position this person is even taking on this topic.' But then I start feeling guilty about it, thinking that I am a bad person for not caring about this topic or that I am rude for not listening. Other thoughts also run around in my head, some of which say, make sure you pay attention or people will know you are not interested in this and you will get in trouble for that later. Or don't let this person think you are not interested in their topic because you need this person to listen to you and care about your topic when it comes time for you to speak.'"

Kelsey started to giggle and I could tell this example, as goofy as it was, was resonating with her. She leaned forward and asked, "so where is the authenticity in all of this?"

"The authenticity is that I don't care about the topic and I don't agree with the position that is being taken." I replied. "Those are my authentic feelings and my truest self. Everything else going on in my head – all that chatter about what I should or should not think or feel – is nothing more than a big 'ole mind fuck."

Kelsey sat abruptly back in her chair and frantically looked around the coffee shop to see if anyone had heard me say the word, fuck. It always bothered her when I said that word and I decided to capitalize on this situation to explore another example of authenticity.

"Kelsey, tell me what you were just feeling and thinking just right now when you sat upright abruptly?"

"Huh?", she responded looking quizzically toward me.

"Please share with me what you were just feeling and thinking a little while ago when you sat upright abruptly...you know, after I said the word, 'fuck'?"

Kelsey's hazel eyes flashed another panicked look but this time she didn't look around the coffee shop to hear who heard me. She hesitated a moment, took another sip of her latte and responded.

"I was thinking how much I dislike the 'f' word, how violent a word that I feel it is and then I was worried that someone else might have heard it and be judging you as a vulgar person for saying it so I was looking around the room to see who else heard it and who may be judging you."

"Excellent!" I responded. Kelsey's now very wrinkled brow appeared to be wondering if I had really lost it so I quickly continued.

"Your thoughts and feelings about the 'f' word are genuine and true. You are being fully authentic in how you view that word. In the four years I have known you however, I have never until now asked you what you thought about that word and you have never told me. Why is that?"

Kelsey was in a full frown now. "I didn't want to insult you. I know you love the 'f' word and I didn't want to insult you by telling you how degrading of a word I think it is."

As Kelsey's words landed on my ears, inside my chest, I felt my heart sink. I felt that kind of chest pain you feel when you just realized you have been hurting someone you love with out even knowing it. I bowed my head for a moment to gain my composure and also to pray for just the right words.

"Kelsey, I am so sorry that I have hurt you from my use of the 'f' word. I am so grateful to you for sharing your thoughts and feelings around my use of the word. You are showing up in authenticity by expressing your thoughts and feelings around my use of the word. However, looking around to see who else heard it because you are concerned about their judgment of me may not be authentic. You may be concerned about my image or you may be concerned about being judged for keeping company with someone who uses the 'f' word. The reason doesn't matter in this moment. What matters in this moment is that we begin, moment-by-moment, to discern what is our authentic selves and what is not. And as we discern this, then we move onto seeing how it aligns with the agenda of what we want or how it aligns with other's agendas."

I could see that Kelsey was pondering whether she was being authentic for having looked around the room to see who else heard me curse, so I encouraged her to join me in re-visiting the earlier example of the meeting. The point that I was trying to make here was three-fold. First, I was explaining that my thoughts and feelings were authentic but I was feeling guilty for having them. Guilt isn't an authentic feeling – it is what comes when I have a concern for looking good or a concern for pleasing others. The feeling of non-interest and then disagreement with the position were strong feelings of mine and they were authentic. Telling myself that I shouldn't feel that way is guilt. Guilt is inauthentic and it is simply a waste of energy. It would be far wiser use of my energy to use in an inquiry process to explore why I am not interested and why I am in such disagreement with my colleague's position. Furthermore, I could use the inquiry process to explore how I could connect my authenticity with their agenda so as to offer genuine understanding and support should it be my role to do so.

Second, exploring why I am not interested in my colleague's topic and why I am in such disagreement with my colleague's position opens up the possibilities for me to tap into my authenticity and find a genuine connection with my colleague's point of view. There is no guarantee after self-exploration that I will find this genuine connection with my colleague. However, what I do know is that without the exploration, I am likely not to find a genuine connection at all.

Third, the other messages that were running around in my head, such as the ones that told me to make sure I pay attention or people will know I am not interested in this and I will get in trouble for that later, or don't let this person think I am not interested in their topic because I need this person to listen to me and care about my topic when it comes time for me to speak - all these are also inauthentic. I am making up stories in my head about what other people may be thinking and as I do this, I am moving farther and farther away from my authenticity and further into game-playing. As I move into game-playing, I am engaging in covert and overt manipulative behavior to advance my own agenda. It is all inauthentic game-playing and the appearance of respect isn't respect at all; it is manipulation, coercion, and ultimately complete disrespect.

"It is just ridiculous." I announced triumphantly at the end of my long monologue.

I could tell Kelsey was listening and I could also tell she had more questions.

"I get the difference in these examples between being authentic and not. But I don't get how I can remain authentic when others are asking me to play games. How do I nurture my creative self when I have to work within an environment that fully doesn't recognize my gifts?"

"Dang, you are asking some great questions girlfriend!"

Kelsey's calling me out on my use of the 'f' word made me very aware of how much I cuss. In that moment, I wasn't sure if my cussing came from a place of authenticity or a place where I stored my armor – the armor that protected me from feeling all that I often felt or at least I told myself that my armor protected me from feeling. I was wondering in that moment if the cussing had become part of the armor. I knew that would be something to explore later. And now, I certainly knew how my cussing affected Kelsey so, I could hold off on that out of deep and genuine respect for Kelsey. For now, I wanted to return back to the conversation at hand.

"For me Kelsey, it is the difference between recognizing my authenticity and recognizing the agenda on the table. What I mean is that as I am just learning to walk in my own authenticity, I prefer to show up as my authentic self. Yet there are many times when I am caught up in the agenda that is on the table. I don't mean a meeting agenda, I mean that which I feel people are asking from me or that which I am asking of them. My getting caught up in the 'agenda' gets me lost in the agenda and I find myself losing my authentic self for the sake of the agenda. Other times, I can walk away from having engaged in the agenda and have been fully my authentic self. There are very few times, because I feel I am so new at this that I can maintain my authenticity and move fully within the agenda."

"I need another example." Kelsey announced firmly setting her chin on her hands, elbows on the table, leaning forward in a way that really didn't typify her usual graceful lady-like sensibilities. The look of it made me smile in complete amusement. She looked so relaxed – a complete one-eighty from the moment I first met her for our coffee date now almost 45 minutes ago.

"Well, the best example I can give you is a personal one and then I can give you a work one where I didn't show up so well. Remember, I am learning what I teach here so bare with me. Cool beans?"

"Cool beans," Kelsey replied, smiling, still leaning fully relaxed, chin on her hands, elbows on the table.

"OK, so the personal one is a little tough but here goes. You know how much I love Ruben and you know that he has asked for a committed dating relationship?"

Kelsey nodded awkwardly as her chin was still resting in her hands.

"Well, my telling him that I needed to explore what it was that would allow me to make a commitment to him was my way of honoring my authenticity while acknowledging his agenda for a committed relationship. I authentically don't feel peaceful about making a commitment to him even though there are absolutely no red flags, not even yellow ones about who I understand him to be. He is absolutely beautiful. Still, I am not at peace with that decision. He keeps asking and asking for a commitment – which is his agenda - and I keep telling him that I am still doing the exploration into what I would need to be in order to commit to him. I don't accept the feeling of any pressure from him. And I don't accept the notion of any obligation toward him. I am communicating all this to him, which allows me to be authentic while acknowledging the agenda he has placed before me. Is that a helpful example?"

Kelsey emphatically nodded and this time her chin slid out of her hands falling heavily between them. We both giggled aloud at her clumsiness. She leaned back gracefully and pulled her latte near her.

"I understand this example, but aren't you afraid he will get impatient with waiting for you to figure out what you need in order to say yes and decide not to date you?"

"Afraid?" Now I was sitting back in my chair with my eyebrows raised. "Afraid? No. Do I recognize that is a possibility? Yes. But I am not afraid of his making that choice because I am not playing games with him. I am being as honest and true to myself as I know how to be. And because of that, there is no fear. I trust that the right outcome will occur in time."

I felt that warm fuzzy feeling come over me as I responded to Kelsey's question. It was an odd feeling yet, it was a good one.

"Kelsey, I have to thank you. If you hadn't asked me these questions, I wouldn't have realized something I really needed to discover."

"What's that?" Kelsey prodded with a bit of amusement in her voice.

"I wouldn't have realized that being authentic - walking in my truth, feeling my true feelings without reasoning or rationalizing them away - really leads to peace. I mean, I just realized, after talking to you about the situation with Ruben, that I am not fearful of what he may decide as I inquire into why I am not willing to commit to him. If I was rationalizing something or lying to myself or playing some sort of stupid game, than I would be worried. But I am not worried. I trust that authenticity will lead to the choice that is true for me. How cool is that?"

"Way cool Marilee. Now just translate all that into my work life, will you?" Kelsey replied with a mix of sarcasm and grateful compassion.

"Mmmm, yeah... I hear you. OK, I'll share a work example. I was at a conference the other day and a colleague who I respect and adore asked me to serve on a very important national task force. I was so honored by the invitation and I respect this person so very much. I even feel that I 'owe' him a service or two if you know what I mean. I mean, he has done a great deal for me and my career, he is one of those amazing people that you feel like you should do anything that he asks of you because he has given so much to you. Well, that is how I feel about him. However, when he asked me to serve on this committee, it just didn't resonate with me. I mean, the purpose of the task force — it just wasn't what I felt led to be spending my time doing. So, I could genuinely tell him how honored I was to be asked. I could genuinely thank him for asking me and then I told him that the work of the task force was of no interest to me."

"Holy Moses Marilee. Are you kidding me? You said it just like that? How did he respond?" Kelsey was so shocked, she had knocked her latte cup over. But neither one of us hurried to stand her cup upright. Fortunately, it was empty. She had finished it almost 20 minutes ago.

I smiled and replied. "Well, I think I used more words than that. And I hope I was compassionate and honoring when I told him of my response. But I did tell him that the work he proposed did not resonate with me. He looked at me in complete shock and as he did so, I could begin to feel my mind kick in and start some sort of story about how I better think of something quick and change my mind and blah, blah, blah. You know the routine. But instead, I prayed for wisdom and it came. I told him what I felt my work was about now and why his generous offer didn't resonate with me, even though I was sincerely honored by his invitation to me. I also told him what I would be happy to do to serve him should those opportunities arise. As I spoke, he softened and a smile returned to his face. I could see that he was hearing me, that he was understanding me, and I couldn't help think that it was all because I was showing up authentically. But perhaps it was also because he was keeping his own ego in check. I don't really know. I am just grateful that it was a beautiful conversation."

"Wow," Kelsey replied. At some point in my explanation, her jaw had dropped and it was still hanging open even after her initial exclamation. "Well," she continued her jaw drawing now to close. "Either he recognized your authenticity or he thinks you are just simply fucking crazy."

We both burst into laughter at the potential truth of Kelsey's words and her use of the 'f" word. As our laughter died down and our conversation returned to all that we needed to get done that night, we decided we had better bring our beautiful time together to an end and head back to work. We embraced with one of those 'that was a great conversation and I love you dearly for it' hugs and parted ways.

As I drove to my home office, my favorite place to write and grade papers, I thought about how authentic I was being when I cursed. I didn't know the answer to that question. I decided to pay attention to how I felt the next time those words came out of my mouth. Did they bring me peace? Or did they bring me anxiety? Did I need to justify them, or explain them, or rationalize their use? If so, I was not being authentic. I smiled at the thought of my doing this. And my smile widened with the joy of the thought of being authentic. I recognized that I had a long journey ahead of me; a long journey to the center of my authenticity; to the center of my greatness. But there, there I would find no more need to hide who I am and who I am becoming. There I would be able to nurture others into their authenticity and into their greatness. And there, there in the center would be pure peace, love, and joy, right there in the center of being, in the center of greatness.

As I pulled into my garage celebrating these new found thoughts of joy and peace and greatness, my phone rang. It felt as if it was an alarm. It was my dear friend, Juan, calling from his home in Boston.

"Hey Juan, how is it going?" I joyfully answered as I sprang from my Jeep, delighted and grateful to have arrived home safely; something I no longer took for granted after watching evening after evening television news of other human beings getting unexpectedly blown to pieces in the midst of simply going about their day-to-day.

"Do you have a minute, I really need to ask you a question?" Juan replied rather hurriedly and quite unlike the normal laid back, fully present conversations I so value and that I typically have with him over the phone.

"Sure", I said, "No problem. What's up Juan?" I pulled my way too tightly stuffed briefcase from the passenger side of the Jeep, set it down on the garage floor, hit the button to close the garage door and walked up the steps to my living room to find a quiet seat on my couch. I realized from the tone of his voice that I would need to be fully present for this conversation. As I sat down on my comfy earth-tone couch, Juan began.

"What do you do when you are in a relationship with someone you love and they seem to have issues with your greatness?" His voice was stern and steady yet I couldn't help detect a note of urgency in his tone. I glanced down at my watch to see that it was just after 6:35 p.m. my time; that was 9:35 his time, *he couldn't be in a meeting right now. Or could he?*

"Huh?" I said, "I don't get what you are asking Juan. I am sorry, I am not following you. Can you re-state the question differently?"

"Sure," he replied. "I noted that the urgent tone in his voice did not subside. "It's Karlina," he said his voice raising in anxiety. "I don't think she understands what I had to sacrifice to get where I am in my career. What do you do when that happens?"

I could feel my brow furrow. I was fully perplexed.

"I am sorry Juan. I still don't get what you are asking. Do you feel Karlina does not understand what your job is about and how it connects with the way you make meaning? Or is she asking you not to shine in your greatness?"

I have no idea why I asked these questions. Perhaps it was because I was aware of who Juan is and how powerful he shows up. His presence often intimidates others, not because he intends to do so, but because his confidence, his integrity, his authentic genuineness is often more than what many folks are accustomed to seeing. Or perhaps it was because I knew how much he loved Karlina and the long distance relationship that he was enjoying with her was beginning to stress his ability to compartmentalize his time with her, with his son, and at his job.

Juan was silent in response to my question. So I glanced down at the phone to see if we were still connected. As I did so, I heard a faint response and I quickly pulled the phone back up to my ear.

"I guess I mean, how do I manage her being OK with my greatness?" Juan said rather sheepishly. I could tell, even from a distance that he was feeling sad, disappointed, and increasingly self-conscious about the questions and perhaps even the circumstances, of which I didn't know anything about, that may have led him to call me.

"You don't." I said with an abruptness that jolted my body upright. I had shocked my own body with the words that came loudly and forcefully from my mouth. Apparently I had shocked Juan as well for there was no response.

Worrying about whether I would lose the opportunity to hear his response should I pull the phone away from my ear and see if he was still there, I instead, pressed it more tightly to my ear almost as if to squeeze a response from him.

"I don't *what* Marilee?" He finally replied.

"You don't manage her Juan. Her response to your greatness is not yours to manage. That is hers to own. I mean… think of it Juan, you have to manage how people perceive your greatness at work, making sure they are not threatened by your brilliance, your creativity, your integrity, and the power of your genuineness. You have to do that every single day so that others feel they can shape the agenda on the table. You have to down play your greatness at work every day while others are taking the time to build their own confidence, build their own genuine knowing about their abilities, their acceptance of what they are and are not. You have to down play your magnificence until they choose to recognize theirs and step into their greatness. Once they do, once people around you step into their greatness, then there is a mutual recognition that neither of you have to down play who you are and are not nor down play who you are becoming. You can just be who you authentically are and that allows others to shine as who they are and are not. All is well in authenticity land. There is no need to manage anyone or anything."

I could hear Juan stifle a laugh at my remark about authenticity land but it didn't slow me down. I was so passionate about this topic having just come from the conversation with Kelsey at the coffee shop. And I knew this conversation with Juan was no coincidence. It was an opportunity for me to seal my learning.

"Juan, do you really want to bring the need to manage your greatness into your personal life, especially when you have to do it so much at work? Wouldn't you rather invite your personal life to be about mutually nurturing each other into your individual and connected greatness and a mutual commitment to facilitating all that you are becoming and all that you are not becoming as individuals and as a couple?"

Again, I heard a silence. I chose to look down at the phone this time. I realized I had talked an awfully long time. All bars were showing, so I pulled the phone quickly back to my ear to make sure I wouldn't miss hearing Juan's thoughts.

"I love her Marilee. I don't know how to support her in being OK with who I am when I am fully shining in my authenticity; when I have the opportunity to demonstrate the power that I have been blessed with and it is fully shining through to others. I don't know how to make her feel comfortable in those moments." His voice sounded desperate and now I began to understand why his sense of urgency had been there before. He so desperately wanted to fix how she felt and he didn't know how to do it because it wasn't his to fix.

"Juan, just as badly as you would like for Karlina to feel comfortable within her own skin as you shine as the one you are created to be, so must you feel at peace being the one you are created to be without regard for how comfortable she feels with that. What I mean is that you don't ignore how she feels. You can talk about it and use inquiry to determine whether there is some aspect of you that she feels is inauthentic as you shine. That would be a great opportunity to explore. Similarly, you can discuss with her, using inquiry and not judgment, why it is that she may feel uncomfortable with you as you shine? Is she choosing to feel unworthy of you? If so, from where does that unworthiness originate? Is she resentful that life circumstances have not provided her with the same opportunities you have had to become great? If so, why is it that she is choosing resentment, rather than joining you in celebration and then seeking how to co-create new similar opportunities for herself now or in the future? I have no idea what the conversation can be between you and Karlina, so use your beautiful wisdom and explore the possibilities without judgment. Is that helpful wonderful Juan?" I was exhilarated by the conversation for as I spoke, new awareness with regard to my inability to commit to Ruben was coming to me.

"I think so Marilee. I will give it a try and keep you posted. Thank you dear friend." He spoke softly and the urgency and anxiety appeared to leave his voice.

"It is my honor brilliant Juan. Your questions have provided me with new insight into my own situation. Thank you, dear friend." I replied with gratitude and felt warm tears begin to stream down my cheek.

We concluded with a few general comments and then we hung up after affirming our love for one another.

Upon ending the call, I went back down to the garage, pulled my heavy briefcase onto my shoulder and made my way back toward the comfy earth-tone grounding couch. I set my briefcase on the floor next to the couch and pulled my journal out. I began to write.

I now know why I am not committing to Ruben. I am simply not comfortable in my skin when I am with him. There is nothing to fix about that, there is nothing to explore about that. He is beautiful as he is and is not. I am beautiful as I am and am not. But as a pair? No, not comfortable. I didn't feel a connectedness for nurturing greatness as a couple. I felt him nurture my greatness and I felt I nurtured his, but it felt so very individual. I will call him tomorrow and let him know that I see nothing but beauty in him, yet he is simply not the one for me. I don't have to make a story up about it. It just is. No judgment, no drama, just is.

I placed the journal on the coffee table and leaned back on the couch. A warm affirming sense of peace rushed over my entire body. I closed my eyes and imagined how it would be if people all over the world recognized just how amazing they were each individually created to be. It was a vivid image I saw. There were no yellow smiley-faced balloons floating around or multi-colored rainbows painting the sky. I did see, however, people who were walking in their power – their power to love, to bring peace and empowerment to others, to nurture their individual and collected greatness and to find solutions to problems of the present while creating innovations to prevent the problems of the future.

No one needed to hide who they really were in this vision. People were authentically showing up – some feeling more empowered than others and others empowering folks into their own gloriousness. There was no one belittling another or becoming defensive because they felt attacked for having a different opinion or a different way of being. No one felt misunderstood, rather all felt seen, fully seen for no one was wearing any armor – there simply wasn't any need for armor that protected against verbal exchanges. There was no need for armor that kept out love and kept people from fully being seen for who they are and who they are becoming. There was no violence, no judgment, no need to fear whether one would be blown up on the way to the grocery store or on his way home from work.

The vision was, well… way cool. It was peaceful, and joyful, and I could feel (I gotta say it) the love; love for oneself and each other. It was gorgeous – simply gorgeous.

CHAPTER NINETEEN

Pause and Integrate

"Seriously, I am telling you. I learned this on the yoga mat first and now I am applying it to my life. I think I have to show it to you in order for you to get what I am trying to say." I was adamant about my announcement to Loretta.

Loretta and I were taking one of my favorite morning walks along the Pacific Beach (PB) boardwalk in San Diego however, this time, we were walking in the early evening instead of in the morning, when there are far less people on the boardwalk.

"I don't get it Marilee. I don't get what you are talking about." Lorettta responded and I could feel her growing frustration.

I stopped in mid-stride, convincing her to walk with me over to the little patch of grass that was nearby so I could physically demonstrate what I had been talking about. Yes, we were both hesitant to walk over onto the little patch of grass because, well… for one, it was a very small patch of grass. We had seen many, many people sprawled out on it doing all sorts of disgusting things and two, I didn't have a yoga mat with me to serve as a buffer between the place where disgusting things occurred and where my body would be practicing yoga.

"I don't think this is a very good idea Marilee. Why don't we just wait until tomorrow to continue this conversation?" Loretta nervously asked, looking around onto the patch of grass, the concrete that surrounded it, and the many passer-bys who were bumping into her as she stopped to watch me make my way onto the grassy area. Her anxiety in her voice grew as she saw the determination in my eyes and in my body.

"No, no, this is too important. This is what the entire concept is based upon. I need to show you." I exclaimed as I literally drug Loretta by the arm to position her in what I thought would be a safe place as I positioned myself on the little patch of grass along the Pacific Beach boardwalk.

Loretta and I often wonder which one of the two of us is the most stubborn. In this moment, I was clearly demonstrating that I was the winner of Ms. Stubborn USA.

I got to the patch of grass where Loretta could stand safely from the sidewalk and view my actions. I have to admit that I did pause to make sure there was nothing identifiably disgusting before removing my shoes and moving onto my hands and knees.

I was explaining to Loretta that Baron Baptiste [27] teaches the principles of yoga to be viewed as the foundation of our yoga practice and once we establish those foundational principles, we can be in the asanas, which embody them while moving carefully into new asanas, asanas that might challenge our growth even more. It is, as Baron Baptiste describes it, the notion of "pause and integrate."

To demonstrate this notion, I came to my hands and knees, hip's width apart, and in table-top position; meaning that my hands were also on the ground, shoulder's width apart. As I was in this table-top position, I was explaining to Loretta that one of the principles of yoga is alignment of joints as well as an elongation of the spine. In addition, I wanted to make sure my shoulders were rolled back and relaxed and that I had a firm foundation with my knees and hands. Other principles include the ujjayi breathing; a diaphragmatic, oceanic sound-like breathing through a closed mouth. More importantly, in the style

---

27　Baptiste, B. (2004). 40 Days to Personal Revolution: A Breakthrough Program to Radically Change Your Body and Awaken the Sacred Within Your Soul. New York, NY: Fireside.

of yoga that Baptiste teaches, the use of breath is extremely important; it is literally one breath with one movement. This was one of my favorite yogic principles for it encouraged mindfulness and full body, mind, and spirit integration.

While I was demonstrating table-top pose, I was clueless to the audience that was gathering around me. Had I been demonstrating this yoga pose at 9:00 a.m. in the morning, there would have been no audience. However, at 6:00 p.m. on a Thursday evening, I was gathering an audience.

Visitors to PB were accustomed to evening street entertainers, semi-professional and professional. They were also accustomed to seeing average Joe's just do "weird" things. I was apparently and un-noticeable to me quickly falling into the latter category.

When I finally did notice the gathering crowd – mostly from Loretta nervously glancing around as I attempted to make eye contact with her - I didn't care. I was determined to make a point with Loretta that there are fundamental principles to yoga practice that are used in any position or asana. Through daily practice, these principles become so embedded into how we do yoga that when new asanas are introduced into the practice (especially new asanas that challenge us to grow in our practice), the new becomes an integration into existing foundational principles, rather than an addition of something that then finds the body out-of-balance, or in shock, or in pain as a result of trying something new.

I explained to Loretta that Baron had led us through the practice where we went from table-top to downward dog to dolphin pose to fore-arm headstand. [28]I demonstrated these asanas as I spoke to

---

28 Downward dog is a pose that you can move into from table-top pose by simply using core strength to gently lift the buttocks toward the sky while keeping the hands on the floor. The idea is to move into downward dog with no stress to the lower back while keeping the head dangling down in a relaxed manner, shoulder blades rolled back and down. The body may look like an inverted "V" when the posture is completed.

Dolphin pose is downward dog except now you are scooting your feet closer to your arms and placing your forearms down onto the ground. You want to maintain the inverted "V" position with your body, along with

Loretta, all the while ignoring the crowd that was increasing in size. As I demonstrated moving into these asanas, I explained to Loretta how each asana, while seemingly new, was built on the same yoga principles of foundation, breath, alignment, and elongation of spine. While it appeared that I was moving into a new pose, one after the other, all I was really doing was integrating new movement into the foundation that had been established in the stability of table-top pose. I also explained how I was using the breath to ease the integration process mindfully. The breath removed any struggle or forcing. The presence of breath just allowed it all to happen with ease and grace.

As I was standing on my head, legs straight up in the air in fore-arm headstand, I could hear Loretta's begging tone in her voice.

"I got it now Marilee. Thanks so much, you can get down now."

"No, wait Loretta, there is more. This is where the lesson really landed in me." I explained with my legs straight up in the air.

"As I was breathing deeply in this asana – breathing deeply in fore-arm headstand - Baron told us to bend at our knees so that our ankles and feet move in front of our heads. In essence, he was coaching us to slowly move into a back bend and then into wheel position.[29] I immediately thought he was insane. There was no way I was going to be able to do that. But then he reminded us that all we had to do when faced with a new challenge on our mat is to pause and integrate. The same principles, the same mindfulness that got us into forearm

---

relaxed and rolled back shoulder blades while your forearms are now on the ground.

Forearm stand can be reached from dolphin by slowly moving your legs closer and closer to your forearms and then lifting the legs, one at a time, so that your legs are in the air and you are balancing only on your forearms. It is a gorgeous asana and the only way I can get into it is if I focus fully on relaxing my breathing and allowing the balance to occur. If I am anxious, or if I work at getting into forearm stand, I immediately fall out of it. If I focus on my breath and simply lift my legs, I can stay in it easily for 10-15 breaths.

29 Wheel position is basically a back bend where your hands and feet are firmly planted on the floor but your back is facing down. You can think of it as a reverse table-top position in some fashion, except that the fingers of the hands face toward your feet rather than away from your feet.

headstand would get us into wheel from forearm headstand. So, he coached us to pause and integrate as we moved forward."

As I was explaining this all to Loretta, I was still, oddly enough, holding the asana of forearm stand on the little patch of grass. I could hear Loretta gasp as I began to bend my knees so that my feet were now dangling just above my head. I explained to Loretta, while I was in this bent forearm stand, that I could feel the stress of the compression on my lower back so I paused and integrated elongation, alignment, breath, and foundation into this new place of being. As I did so, the compression disappeared and I was just as comfortable there – on my forearms, with my knees bent, feet dangling in front of me - as I had been in table-top position. However, when Baron coached us into placing our feet down onto the ground and moving into wheel, I froze. I told myself I couldn't do it. I told myself that this was as far as I was going today.

Just as I was convincing myself to come out of the bent legged forearm stand, one of Baron's Master teachers came by and literally squatted down to look into my face. She smiled a bright, glowing smile, and she told me to first believe that I could do it, and then breathe into setting my feet down onto the ground. She told me I could move as slowly as I wanted to, integrating the newness of the asana into every breath I took. Her smile was convincing and so was her tone. However, I was still not moving. I seemed to have been stuck in my "pause". In my "stuckness," I saw the beautiful Master teacher's smile straighten. She was now quite stern. All she said in a very authoritative voice was,

"Marilee, you have to let go of that which is making you hold your pause, so you can integrate that which is new into your practice."

They were words of magic. I "let go" of my not believing I could do it. I breathed and integrated the foundational principles as I experienced the newness of setting my feet down to the ground behind my head. When there, I paused, returned to the basics and then straightened my arms. I had moved from table-top to a full wheel via a forearm headstand. I felt on top of the world. I jumped up screaming a big "yes" aloud. And just as in Baron's boot camp, the crowd there, as it did here on the Thursday evening in Pacific Beach, gave me noticeable verbal encouragement.

I looked up at Loretta after standing to my feet. I had forgotten she was there. I was so into my pause and integrate mode, recalling the profound lesson that had been taught to me, that I had forgotten I was sharing it with her. Her jaw was dropped and her eyes looked wildly open, yet alert and attentive. I smiled a huge smile when my eyes met hers. And she ran over to me, throwing her arms around me exclaiming how amazing that just was. I laughed so hard we almost fell over onto the patch of green, with which we previously had been trying so hard to avoid making contact. Laughing to ourselves, unconcerned whether the on-lookers thought we were crazy, we moved back into our walk.

"So, does that make sense now?" I asked Loretta so excited about having had the opportunity to demo it to her in person.

She nodded, "I get what it looks like on the mat, but tell me again what it looks like off the mat."

"Of course," I replied so excited to return to our conversation brushing little pieces of grass off my forearms.

"And that is Baron's point by the way; he stresses that we need to practice yoga on the mat so that we can carry its principles off the mat. But I digress..."

I explained to Loretta that for me, pause and integrate was exactly what I had been missing from my life. When something new came along, it often consumed me. It didn't matter whether it was a job, a project at work, a project at home, a new relationship; I simply became consumed with it. And then when the consumption period was over, I would look at it like it was some type of foreign object that I didn't know with what to do. Integration, particularly the pausing part and the mindful breathing, allowed me to conscientiously integrate that which was new into the foundational being of who I am, how I move, and what I value. The principles of pause and integrate allowed me to check in with my foundation; that which was my source power, that which gave me strength. And it didn't matter whether what was new was welcomed or unwelcomed. It didn't matter whether it was an exciting new relationship or a new 5 plus centimeter growth in my right ovary that wasn't there a month ago. I could pause and integrate it into who I am and who I am becoming. I could breathe as I did so and when I did, my foundation never shook.

Loretta walked in silence while I spoke and when I finished, she was still silent. I respected her silence and then remembered that there was one more important aspect of all this that I had forgotten to share.

"Loretta?"

"Hmm," she responded. I knew I had disturbed her from deep thoughts.

"I am sorry I disturbed you from your thoughts, but I need to tell you about the other key piece of all of this for me. Is that OK?" I had stopped walking and had turned to face her. The sun was setting but there was still plenty of light. The street lamps had not yet come on.

Loretta stopped walking as well and turned to face me. Her eyes looked distant. I wasn't sure she had heard anything I was sharing yet, I felt that she had and was just in the deep place of processing that she often needed to be after hearing things that were new in concept to her.

"Go ahead Marilee, what is it?" She smiled slightly as she encouraged me to continue. And so I did.

"Do you remember me telling you the part where Baron's Master teacher told me to let go?"

She nodded silently in reply.

"Well, Loretta, that is a big part of pause and integrate. I realized I had to let go of the belief that I couldn't integrate the new asana into my foundational principals in order to move forward into wheel. I also had to let go of the belief that it would hurt. I didn't know that it would hurt. It was new so I thought it would hurt. Letting go of the belief that you can't integrate what is new to you or that it will hurt if you do is a huge part of the pause and integrate process. Does that make sense?"

Loretta nodded and I could see tears coming to her eyes. I wasn't sure why the tears were there but in this moment, I wasn't going to ask. I was going to let go of the need to question and to understand.

Instead, I put my arms around her, gave her such a tight squeeze that I heard her gasp for air. Apologizing for squeezing her so tightly, I immediately released her from my hug and she slid gently out of my embrace. She started laughing and teased me about needing to let go of my need to hug so tightly so I could better integrate our friendship into her delicate frame. We laughed aloud and strolled on down the boardwalk in silence.

"I think I get it," Loretta announced to the ocean a short while later. "I think I get the pause and integrate concepts. Now, all I need to do is let go of the fear of that which is in front of me so that instead of resisting it, I can integrate it firm into my foundation, firm within my principles, and knowing that my source of power will prevail."

I smiled as I looked at Loretta who never made eye contact with me during her pronunciation. We just continued to walk in silence. She made me think as she always does. Letting go can consist of letting go of that which consumes us or that which we resist. Either way, in order to pause and integrate, we need to let go. And determining what we need to let go of isn't really that hard. I am either afraid of it or consumed by it. But whatever it is, it is there right in front of me or beside me or trailing closely on my heels. Time to pause and integrate it into the firm foundation that rests on my source power. Nothing can rock that, as long as I remember to breathe.

CHAPTER TWENTY

Accepting Acceptance

"I disagree," I exclaimed placing the bottle of Vancouver, British Columbia pinot noir down after pouring a glass and then pushing it down the counter towards Susanna. "I don't think accepting something is a passive practice at all."

"How can it *not* be passive?" Susanna exclaimed, stopping the sliding bottle with such grace and finesse, as if we were shooting a beer commercial in a western saloon. "Acceptance is for those who don't have the guts to fight."

"Good catch." I interrupted her argument genuinely impressed with her style and the ease at which she caught the bottle I had slid rather forcefully toward her down my long granite counter top. "I see you accepted that bottle with style and grace."

Susanna laughed a lyrical, hearty laugh and responded with a sarcastic retort. "Accepting this fine bottle of wine is a pleasure, it needs very little consideration or action. I just reached out and grabbed it as it was passing by."

My eyes lit up as Susanna spoke. "Isn't reaching out and grabbing that bottle action?"

Susanna laughed, "I see what you are getting at Marilee; it *is* action, but it is not a very difficult act. It is more of a reaction, I think. I *wanted* the bottle of wine that was passing in front of me."

"Ooh, good point," I responded rather excited about how this example was just emerging for both of us. "Accepting something can be reactionary, just as not accepting it can be reactionary. You could have just as easily responded in a manner that knocked the bottle off the counter. You could have done that just as easily as the action that grabbed the bottle and pulled it closer to you. Neither action or reaction required much effort but the action you chose required your consideration and then a choice. Didn't it? Or am I just talking to hear the sound of my voice?"

Susanna giggled. She seemed to be just as amused with the organic emergence of our example as I was. "You often talk to hear the sound of your voice but this time… I think this time is an exception. I get your point. However, accepting a fine bottle of wine at 7:18 p.m. on a Saturday night requires very little consideration. It was almost passive."

Susanna held up her left hand to hold off my verbal retort. She paused just a moment to pour herself a glass from the bottle she was still clutching in her right hand and then she continued.

"Accepting that you have cancer or that you have been raped or that you lost your job or that your husband cheated on you for the fifth time…you get my point… *that* my friend…accepting *that*… Well that, THAT is for the passive folks, the folks who don't have the guts to fight."

I stared at Susanna as she swirled her glass of wine on the granite counter top. I watched her face. It looked as it held a mixture of smugness for having "won" the debate with which we were just engaged and it also held pain, fear, sorrow, and anger. No where on her face did I see joy, peace, or even a glimpse of happiness. No where. It didn't even appear when she took her first sip after carefully swirling the wine, sniffing it, swirling it again, and then taking the ever so light sip of air as you bring the wine to your lips and take it onto your taste buds. I stared at her while she took her second sip. I still saw no sign of happiness or joy or peace.

Susanna was lost in her thoughts and lost in tasting the wine. Watching her, I found my mind beginning to consume me and removing me from the end of the counter where I stood in the same room with Susanna.

It now felt as if we were in two separate rooms or two separate worlds. We were lost in our own thoughts, our own memories, and our own questions. I was amazed by how quickly that all transpired and while I understood how to get back into the present moment, I wasn't sure I actually wanted to disturb Susanna. It was as if she needed this time. And maybe she didn't. Either way, I chose to let her be and my mind went back to the words she last spoke.

Her words had taken me back to my past; back to times when all I new how to do was fight. The fighting left me either feeling victorious for trampling some other person's spirit or character or it led to my surrender. However that surrender; that surrender didn't involve any conscience choice of acceptance. That surrender was an exhaustion, an admittance that I could no longer fight. In that surrender, my energy, intellect, and feelings had been used up and dried out and there were no more resources available. There was no reprieve to be seen on the forefront. No one was coming to rescue me or aid me or support me or relieve me. It was a fight to the bitter end and surrender was the option over death.

This new kind of surrender I was exploring, well, this kind of surrender was not for those who didn't have "guts". This surrender required accepting what had happened (whatever it was), accepting how I felt about it and thought about it for what it was and what it was not. As Baron Baptiste [30]taught us, the 100% acceptance of what it was and what it is not must come first. This kind of acceptance required a deep agreement, an agreement of the soul and it required a moment-by-moment choice. It was not a one-time get it out of the way for the rest of your life decision; it was a moment-by-moment acceptance.

And what did I get in return? Expanding energy. Fighting depleted me. Accepting, although not even close to being a passive action, gave me energy. In looking at what I had previously been battling straight

---

30   Baron Baptiste, Founder of Baron Baptiste Power Vinyasa Yoga – www. baronbaptiste.com

in the eyes and accepting it all for what it was and for what it was not, the energy that was spent fighting was mine to use for inquiry; to use for inquiry into what may come as a result of accepting, rather than fighting.

Surrendering now had a new meaning to me. It was not an action that I did as a result of either dying or giving up. It was an action that I chose as a result of accepting what was and what was not. In choosing acceptance of being raped, of having a disease, of being twice divorced, of having tumors growing inside of me, of seeing young men return from war without arms and legs, and of chatting with people who had no home and no job every day… accepting what is and what is not in all of this, even though it was a moment-by-moment choice was not defeat. It was not passive. And each choice of acceptance was certainly filled with plenty of consideration.

Choosing, in this moment to come back into the room where Susanna was, back into the space where she was still swirling and sipping her wine, lost in thought, lost in memory, lost in battle, without any sign of joy on her face, I chose acceptance once again.

"Susanna," I said softly, knowing that the sound of my voice would disturb her from the world she had been occupying in the last few moments. "Susanna," I said again, this time a little louder for she had not appeared to hear me at all the previous time.

"Susanna, accepting rape, or divorce, or cancer is not an acknowledgement of defeat."

Susanna glanced up at me, scowling for a moment and it appeared that she was only scowling because I had been so rude as to pull her out of her own world and back into mine. Realizing that she was scowling, her face softened and she stood a little straighter as if to collect herself for another verbal debate. Yet, she remained quiet. Her gaze returned to her swirling wine glass.

"I recognize that I am not the best one to share for I am still knee deep in learning this lesson myself. But for example, when I accepted my disease for what it is and what it is not, I realized I had a full life to live, even if it meant making adjustments to how I live. Fighting it, refusing to admit that it was what it was and was not was exhausting. But when I accepted it and made adjustments to how I live, those adjustments created more space for me to invest even more into my well-being. I have made more loving decisions in order to enhance my well-being – decisions I never before would have considered. And accepting my rape for what it is and what it *is not* meant I no longer judged myself for what had happened and that created more space to not judge myself in other situations."

Susanna didn't look at me. My words were landing empty on the counter top in front of us both. I asked myself whether I would accept just being with her in her pain and not trying to share the lesson I learned. Perhaps, I should have chosen just accepting being present with her in her pain, but I didn't. My mouth opened and I knew more words were going to spew forth.

"However, once I accepted that I had an addiction to peanut M&Ms, I could see it for what it was and what it was not."

Susanna pulled herself upright abruptly and jerked her head toward me. I could tell she wasn't sure what I had just said. So I repeated myself.

"It's true, once I accepted my addiction, I could move into the inquiry of why I felt I needed peanut M&Ms. I wasn't fighting them anymore and the acceptance gave me energy to ask questions I hadn't asked before and that led to answers that I never thought existed. It was energizing rather than defeating. Does that make sense?"

"You are *crazy* Marilee. Down right crazy." She cocked her hip as she spoke and I began to see a hint of a smile.

Yes, there you are little smile. Welcome back.

I smiled back at Susanna and affirmed to her that the announcement of my insanity was old news. But I explained to her that she may want to try practicing acceptance on something a little smaller than her rape.

"Perhaps you should try practicing it on your addiction to Kenneth Cole boots."

"25 pairs of Kenneth Cole boots is NOT an addiction." She retorted playfully.

"That looks a lot like fighting and very little like acceptance," I playfully chided.

"OK," she said reluctantly. "I'll try it on. I'll try it on with the joy I would try on a pair of Kenneth Cole boots. I'll inquire into why I am addicted to Kenneth Cole books when I go shopping at the outlets tomorrow."

We both laughed at the imagery Susanna had just painted and then moved to the living room where we had planned to watch a chic flick while talking about nothing in particular.

When Susanna left my home for the evening, I replayed our conversation in my head. I wondered if she really would consider acceptance as powerful a tool as fighting. I wondered if the inquiry would open up to her as it did to me when I decided choosing to fight was just getting more of what I already had and nothing of what I didn't have. And I chose to accept beautiful Susanna for all that she is and is not.

CHAPTER TWENTY-ONE

Thank You Jesus

"Why do you say that Marilee?" Miranda questioned as we pulled into a very tight parking space at 9:00 p.m. on a cool Thursday evening. The moon was hidden by the marine layer so the only light we had was the light coming from the surrounding businesses; the street lights were completely out for a reason we didn't know.

"Say what?" I replied somewhat startled from concentrating on trying to fit my Jeep into such a tight parking spot and feeling the fullness of my bladder increasing my need to get to a restroom fairly quickly.

"Why do you thank Jesus whenever you are expressing gratitude? I don't get it. I don't mean to be disrespectful or anything but... I mean, what did Jesus have to do with our finding a parking space in Venice Beach?"

Miranda asked this question with the intense curiosity of a two-year old. I could feel her genuineness in the questioning and I could sense her passion. And...I was shocked to hear the question. I hadn't even realized I had thanked Jesus as we found a parking space. I was so grateful to find one before I peed my pants. It was, upon brief reflection, a great question. One I had actually never been asked before in my entire 46 years on this planet in this set of skin.

"That is a great question Miranda; a great question. Can I answer it after I pee? I am dying here." I didn't wait for Miranda's answer. I was out of the Jeep and headed very quickly into the Rubio's where we were going to empty our bladders, grab a to-go bite to eat, and then get back on the road. We had been doing some work at a near-by institution. It was a great day but a very long day. We were anxious to get home. We were tired and we wanted to sleep in our own beds. We knew we had a good 2 and ½ hour drive ahead of us as long as there was no traffic with which to contend.

As I sprinted into the restroom, I faintly heard Miranda asking what I wanted to eat after declaring that I didn't have to answer the question if I didn't want to do so. I thought about what she asked as I waited in line to use the one toilet in the entire restaurant (we should have known better than to expect a lot of toilet options so close to the beach).

Upon exiting, I noticed that Miranda had ordered for both of us. Without speaking a word to each other, I realized that it was now my job to grab the to-go order and appropriate condiments, utensils, and napkins and meet Miranda back in the car after she was able to make her way through the restroom line.

Once back in the car and after having gratefully reimbursed Miranda for my meal, I repeated Miranda's question. She laughed as she heard me re-state it and said again that I didn't need to answer it if I didn't want to. I assured her that I did because it was a great question, but I wasn't sure how eloquent my answer would be.

"Why do I thank Jesus? That is a really great question Miranda. Thank you so much for asking it, seriously, thank you."

"I just don't understand it Marilee. You are not a Christian, right? So why do you thank Jesus?" Miranda was just as passionate and as intense as she was when she first asked the question.

I giggled in hearing her ask me the question again, but this time, I was sure that it was a nervous giggle, as if to represent my inner fear that I didn't know the answer to her question, rather than a giggle that resonates from a place of amusement. So, I sat back in my driver's seat, took a deep slow breath and prayed for wisdom. I prayed that more than anything, I would be made more mindful of all the words that flowed from my mouth and that they would fully represent the intention that I wanted going out to the Universe. I no longer wanted to waste a single word.

"Miranda, I am grateful to you for asking the question because I realize that I have not been as conscious as I could be when I offer up prayers of gratitude and invitation. Thank you for pointing that out to me."

Miranda replied back rather panicky, "I am not trying to criticize you Marilee, I just want to understand why you say some of the stuff you do. I mean, I don't get it. I consider you an intellectual and here you go thanking some guy in history for finding us a parking place. I don't get it."

I laughed as I heard Miranda speak. I loved how she was boiling down the perspectives of many people into this innocent and genuine conversation. I didn't feel attacked and I didn't feel threatened. I was simply grateful for her questions. For it is through inquiry where I get the opportunity to discover who I am and who I am not and invite in who I am becoming.

"Please don't worry Miranda. I am really grateful for the question. This will be a fun topic to discuss with you on our long ride home. Thank you so much."

I began by explaining to Miranda that first off, to determine whether I was a Christian really depended on one's definition of a Christian. I explained to her that I had this conversation with Karl, as he is a practicing Christian and I am not. What I meant by being a practicing Christian in this context is that he attends a Christian church and participates in a Christian community and I do not – at least not right now. Who knows what the future will hold?

In any event, I explained to her that Merriam Webster defines a Christian as "one who professes belief in the teachings of Jesus Christ or is a member of one of the Churches of Christ separating from the Disciples of Christ in 1906 or one who is a member of the Christian denomination having part in the union of the United Church of Christ concluded in 1961."[31] So, while I am not a member of that church, I do believe in many of the teachings of Jesus. At least I believe in the ones that I understand and can integrate into my day-to-day. I don't understand all that Jesus taught and therefore, for me, it makes it difficult for me to believe in something I don't know how to practice. As a matter of fact, I learned more from what Jesus taught by reading a Buddhist writer, Thich Nhat Hanh, [32]than I learned from untold numbers of Bible studies and Catechism courses.

"Jesus is the great teacher of how to be love Miranda. Buddha is also a great teacher of love as is Ghandi, Thich Nhat Hanh, and Nelson Mandela. And heck, I even learned a lot from John Lennon. Religions have been born out of the teachings of Jesus and Buddha. And there are certainly other religions that have been born from those who teach about love and those who do not. But not all those who are great teachers of Love have born a religious practice as a result of their teachings. So, if to be a Christian is to believe that the teachings of Jesus with regard to how to be love are true, than yes, I am a Christian. If to be Christian means that I belong to one of the formal religious sects that profess Christianity and various interpretations of Jesus' teachings, than it is correct to say that I am not a Christian. Is that helpful?"

"That is helpful." Miranda graciously replied. "But it doesn't answer my question." She smiled at me as she prodded me to continue. I smiled back and assured her that I would answer but I actually needed to clarify her perception of me because I was thinking that a lot of our conversation may get off-track if we don't understand the meaning behind the words we are choosing.

"I thank Jesus, Buddha, the Universe, the Holy Spirit, God, the Creator, the Source...all of these I thank from time-to-time and for me, the names are interchangeable."

Miranda looked up at me in confusion, so I continued.

"What I mean Miranda is – and please forgive how simple I am making this explanation – that these teachers energetically are all the same."

---

31 http://www.merriam-webster.com/dictionary/christian
32 Thich Nhat Hanh, (1995). Living Buddha, Living Christ. New York, NY: Penguin Publishing.

"OK Marilee, now I am really confused." Miranda's nose scrunched up toward her eyes as she made a face of complete frustration. I giggled at the sight of her.

"OK Miranda, let me back up and share something else but forgive me again for over-simplifying everything. Remember that I am teaching what I am learning – cool?"

"Cool." Miranda agreed and her face relaxed as she settled back as best she could into her upright Jeep seat to listen.

"OK, so basically, we live in a world that has micro energy flow called quantum physics and macro energy flow called physics. Let's just say that 'physics' is made up of all the laws that we typically use as we navigate the world we see. For example, physics – the laws that govern the macro world - teaches me that matter can not occupy the same space and time. So, if I was to take my Jeep and try to occupy the same space at the same time that the Mercedes right next to us on the freeway is occupying, I would not be successful. The two objects would crash into each other. That is an example of a macro energy law that governs the world that we see."

"Got it so far." Miranda said encouragingly. "So make sure you stay in your lane. I don't need you to provide an example of that lesson."

Giggling, I continued. "The micro energy world, the world that we don't see, is one we are still discovering and that world is often referred to as the quantum world. [33]Here, we understand that matter can occupy the same space at the same time. We also understand that thoughts are energy and that you can actually influence the flow of energy when you observe it or have intentions behind what you observe. Isn't that cool?"

"Yeah Marilee, it's all cool. I am still waiting for you to answer my initial question." Miranda said again, yet I could sense she was not as impatient as her words would have otherwise led me to believe. I continued with my monologue.

"The point is that I believe that the research emerging from the quantum world is true. I believe there is energy right here in front

---

33 http://physics.about.com/od/quantumphysics/p/quantumphysics.htm

of me – energy that I can not see between my eyes and this steering wheel. The steering wheel is composed of energy that I can see. When I thank Jesus, or God or the Universe, or the Creator, or Buddha, I am thanking the unseen energy that contributes - beyond my ability to see it or comprehend it - to the greater good[34]. For me, God is the unseen energy. Jesus is the unseen energy, even though at one time, Jesus was a great man whom people could see and who ran around his little corner of the earth presenting radical teachings about how to live love and how to be love." I paused a moment to glance at Miranda to see if I was making sense. The way she was looking at me led me to believe I was so I continued.

"Nowadays, for me, Jesus, the former human being, has joined with the unseen energy of the greater good, as has Buddha, who was also a man. They are the unseen energy in that their teachings and those who believe their teachings carry love on energetically and it is often unseen energy as it is exchanged from one to another, even though the acts of love may be seen. Does that make sense?"

Miranda hesitated before responding. "Yes, I understand the physics of which you speak and I believe in those laws as well, even though our understanding of them continues to emerge. It makes sense to me that I can't see the energy of love even though I feel it and even though it may be demonstrated to me in the form of receiving a dozen roses or in Elisa helping me pack up my apartment. But why do you say you thank Jesus and why do you invite God to help you with stuff. Why would you call on something that has nothing to do with what you are doing? I mean, if you want to help a homeless person, get off your ass and buy the homeless person a good meal. If I want to become a full professor, I get off my ass and do the work to become a full professor. Why are you calling on invisible whatever-it-is to help you? That just seems … well… it seems… un–intellectual."

Giggling again in response to Miranda, but this time not from nervousness, from pure amusement, I reassured her that I heard what she was asking and that I was not offended.

---

34 Be sure to refer to earlier references that define prayer and greater good

"These are fabulous questions Miranda. I am so grateful to you. Here is my point. We have a lot of research, and more is being done now, that demonstrates that there are unseen energies that can work to our benefit or not. And we can, if we choose, aid the synergistic coming together of these energies with our thoughts. It is possible, although we don't know for sure, that we can also aid the synergistic coming together of these energies with our words. This makes sense, because typically, thoughts come before words, although I have demonstrated time and time again in my own life that that is not always true."

Miranda let out a howl of laughter that let me know she was fully following my every word, so I continued.

"My speaking messages of gratitude to these unseen energies that I have named Jesus, Buddha, God, the Creator, or the Holy Spirit – all equally interchangeable to me, but I recognize that they are not interchangeable to those around me - means that I am sending out an appreciative acknowledgement to these energies for the role they played in contributing to the greater good. I got to play a physical role in the macro world by seeing the open spot, and driving the physical Jeep into the parking space; I am energetically operating in the world of that which is seen. However, the unseen energy I called Jesus played the role in the world of the unseen by contributing to the seeming coincidence that there just happened to be an open parking spot when I needed it. Some quantum physicists teach that everything operates on a predictable mathematical equation; others feel that it is random yet still possible to define mathematically. Regardless of who is right or wrong - I don't care in this moment - I am simply inviting these unseen energies to assist in creating an open parking space. And whether they did or did not aid in the creation of the open parking space, I am grateful. Is that helpful?"

Miranda lifted one eyebrow and peered at me sideways. "So, you think an unforeseen energy had a role in finding us a parking space at Venice Beach? Are you serious? You found the parking spot. What did the unforeseen energy have to do with it?"

"Well, I don't know, maybe nothing and maybe everything. When we pulled off the interstate, I said a silent pray. I communicated to God (the unseen energy) that I had to go to the bathroom really badly and I prayed for guidance to find a place where we could get both a healthy, quick meal to go and use a clean restroom. Recall that we were looking for parking spots before we were looking for a place to eat and pee and low and behold, there was a parking space available right in front of Rubio's. So, I thanked the unforeseen energy for playing whatever role it may have had in creating that space and I called that energy Jesus. Thus, I thanked Jesus."

Miranda's nose was scrunching up toward her eyes again. "I still don't get it. What did the unforeseen energy have to do with all that?"

"I don't know Miranda, maybe nothing, maybe everything. I am still very grateful for finding a parking spot in the nick of time, which was before my bladder exploded, and I am grateful we also found a healthy quick to-go eating alternative very close to that parking space. I am grateful and instead of keeping the energy of gratitude within me, I let it out via words and named the source of energy to which I was grateful – even though I may have used the 'wrong' name. The point is that I am recognizing in gratitude all that may have helped us get what we needed. And with regard to the greater good, who knows? For now, the greater good is simple – our physical bodies needed both release of waste and nourishment so that we could continue on our journey."

Miranda's face softened again. "OK, I am following you but why did you thank Jesus?"

Smiling and recognizing another reason why Miranda was such a great teacher, I continued. "I could have just as easily thanked God, the Universe, the Holy Spirit, or the Creator. They are all of the same energy source to me. They are all from the center, the core, the original source of all energy. Most of the time I call that energy God. But often, I call it the Holy Spirit, or my Source Power. For me, it is all the same. Again, I recognize that for others, it is not. And this is one of the reasons I am so grateful to you for this conversation Miranda. Without it, I wouldn't know how to perhaps help others understand that when I refer to God in my writing or when I refer to Jesus, they can simply put in the name that has the most meaning to them.'

Miranda remained silent for a while and then spoke softly. "Can you give me one more example?"

"Sure," I said enthusiastically. I was now well aware that I was no longer tired as I was when we stopped for dinner. Recognizing that the healthy food had been good fuel, I was also well aware that this conversation was invigorating and I was so grateful for the clarity that Miranda's questions were providing.

"Remember the book[35] I was reading before my surgery?"

Miranda nodded and replied. "You mentioned that it gave you some great ideas on positively preparing for a successful surgery."

"Yes, it did indeed. Well, the night before the surgery, I prayed to my Source Power; I prayed to God. And in my prayer, with my thoughts, I invited in guidance for me to take a loving perspective on all that I would encounter prior, during - in case I awoke, and after my surgery. I invited in the ability to accept with loving grace whatever the surgeon would discover and I envisioned a successful surgery where I would be walking with Karl on the beach five days after the surgery."

"Yes," Miranda replied reflectively. "I remember you sharing that with us as we drove you to the hospital."

"And do you remember what happened?" I inquired in a manner that now invited her to share her own observations of the lesson I was now intending for us both to learn.

"Yes," Miranda beamed. "First off, the tumors were benign."

With this, I interrupted her. "But Miranda, I didn't pray that I wouldn't have cancer. I prayed that I would lovingly accept all that was discovered and that whatever would happen would serve the greater good. I didn't know that the greater good may be served by my not

---

35 Huddleston, P. (1996) *Prepare for Surgery, Heal Faster: A Guide Of Mind-Body Techniques.* Cambridge, MA: Angel River Press.

having cancer. It could have just as easily been served by my having cancer. I didn't know."

Miranda's nose scrunched up again and I could tell that perhaps I had chosen a bad time to interrupt her. Encouraging her to hold that thought, I asked her to continue.

"Well, I remember that we were laughing all the way to your check-in, and that we got in trouble by another surgeon – not yours of course - for laughing so hard in the pre-op area. I remember meeting your surgical team and asking you how you put all of them together. I remember you telling me you didn't, that God did. And I thought you were just dizzy in the head from the anesthesia and you insisted on telling me you hadn't had any yet. I remember your surgery taking a long time. Elisa and I were really getting nervous. Karl kept calling and we didn't have an update. Then, the surgeon came out. He was so kind and gentle. He told us that it had been a successful surgery, that you were very lucky, and that we should be able to see you in a while. When we finally were allowed back, you were smiling, and offering prayers of thanks. You didn't even know how long you had been under or know whether you had cancer yet. I remember asking if I could have whatever they had put you on because you seemed so at peace and genuinely full of joy."

I laughed in hearty recollection; it was true. When I came to, I didn't know how many slices I had in me, whether I had cancer, or when I would be going home. I was just grateful I had awakened and even though I knew I had pain-killers coursing though my veins, I felt full of joy and peace. I had a confidence that all was well.

I reminded Miranda how she kept saying that everything had turned out just as I had envisioned. We were surrounded with loving caregivers, joyful in their duties and very attentive in their precision. I had undergone a long and very successful laparoscopic surgery, which meant I would be able to go home that night if my bodily functions cooperated, and they did. I still didn't know if the tumors that were removed were benign, but it was highly likely they were benign. And I was very grateful for the prognosis, even though the surgeon let me know that he had to take out both of my ovaries and that he couldn't get all of the diseased tissue.

"The point here Miranda is that I didn't have anything to do with that successful surgery. Yes, I did my part by using my physical form to read that Huddleston book[36] and learn how to invite the non-physical in to aid me in remaining calm prior to surgery and choosing to see everyone and everything as love. You and Elisa also were instrumental in helping. You were there in physical form, which created a solid visual reminder for me about the power of love and that was a great anchor for my positive thoughts and prayers to continue to flow. And you also created more beautiful healing energy because that was your expressed intention to do so. In addition, I had dozens of gorgeous friends and family members praying – sending more positive healing energy my way. I asked the surgical team to read the positive affirmations that I had gotten from the Huddleston book prior to surgery and they did so while holding my hand. I didn't create the successful surgical team or the successful surgery, God did. It was God in the unseen via the prayers and positive thought as well as positive intentions. It was also God in physical form as expressed by the surgeons, nurses, you, Elisa and within me."

"I get it!" Miranda squealed out so loudly that I almost swerved into the next lane of traffic.

"Yeah?" I inquired afraid to say anything. I didn't want to disturb the joy that was resonating from Miranda and flooding the inside of my Jeep.

"Yeah," Miranda affirmed. "I get it. That makes sense to me. But do I have to call the origin of all seen and unseen energy, God? That just doesn't feel right to me."

I smiled softly as I glanced over to her and replied. "Lots of other people don't. Why should you?"

Miranda's face looked peaceful as she settled back into the uncomfortable passenger seat. She looked truly content even though

---

36 Huddleston, P. (1996) *Prepare for Surgery, Heal Faster: A Guide Of Mind-Body Techniques.* Cambridge, MA: Angel River Press.

she couldn't possibly be comfortable in my tattered passenger Jeep seat. I was grateful for Miranda and for the conversation we had just had and so I offered a silent prayer of gratitude to the source energy that I call God (and sometimes I call it Jesus, Buddha, the Holy Spirit, or the Universe).

I was not sure that I had answered her questions fully. I was not sure whether what I had shared was "right." What I shared was what made sense to me; what I shared resonated with me at a high level. What I shared with Miranda was how I understood God and it was how I could best explain how God resides in each one of us and in all that surrounds us. What I shared with Miranda is how I came to believe how all I do see is connected by all that which is unseen and the unseen resides within us and flows through us. It is how I have come to believe that we are all god all of the time. I just really don't know how to teach "it" (e.g., God) and I certainly don't know what to call "it" (e.g., God) but I know "it" is within me and Miranda and everyone we saw today.

I wonder if "it" is concerned with what we call "it". I wonder if "it" cares about how we explain what "it" is. Probably not, because why would "it" care what "it" is called for "it" knows "it" is the One; the true originator of all things seen and unseen; the life source of all seen and unseen. How can we, moving around in the form of the seen, even have an appropriate word for such immense power? How could we possibly name that?

CHAPTER TWENTY-TWO

Being Love or In-Love

"I have no idea." Karl said as he kicked up the sand beneath his feet on the Coronado beach boardwalk. "What do you think it means?"

"I have no idea either. That is why I asked you?" I responded lovingly punching him in the side of his shoulder like a 13-year old would do with a boy upon which she has a crush.

"Well," he said with a slow hint of a southern drawl, looking down at the sand and pausing to play with it, "I guess being in love is the infatuation part of love. I think it may be when two people are caught up in the physical aspect of romantic love and feeling that..."

"...butterflies in your stomach, can't quit thinking about you, you make me wet when I kiss you kind of feeling." I rudely interrupted him but I was so excited that what he was saying was starting to make sense to me, so I couldn't help myself blurt into the conversation.

Karl stopped in his tracks, turned his head towards me half-way, and gave me his classic side grin that, well, gave me butterflies in my stomach, and excitement in my groin and well, you get the picture.

His side grin turned into a full smile as he said, "Yeah, something like that." And then he put his head back down to begin walking again while his feet played in all the sand he could find along the boardwalk.

"Ya know Karl, we could go back to just walking on the beach if ya want." I mentioned to him, as his love for playing in the sand was unavoidably noticeable at the moment.

He gave me his classic half-grin again and without a word, his hand grabbed mine and he pulled me toward the opening where the boardwalk met the beach and we moved closer toward the ocean in silence.

Karl was a tall Norwegian kind of build; probably because his family was from Norway. He was the strong silent type and his wisdom ran deep and wide. He was so easy to hang with; I treasured his company for the peace it brought me and the grounding I felt whenever I was around him. I was enjoying a long weekend of his company and felt so fortunate to have so much time with him. I knew that I loved him and I knew that in light of the fact that I loved many. I just never understood the whole "in-love" versus "love" conversation and I decided that Karl was the perfect person I could ask for the answer. Why? Perhaps partly because he had already taught me so much about relationships and I respected him deeply for his honesty and wisdom. And partly because well, I got warm fuzzy butterflies in my stomach when I thought of him and I was thinking of him way more than what was "normal" for someone that I knew that I loved, whatever that means.

In any event, I wanted to know from him what he thought the difference between being in-love and being loving was; I wanted to understand what being in-love was all about. I really didn't understand it. Love made all the sense in the world to me. But being in love, it seemed that that world was full of jealousy, possessiveness, expectations, and heart-ache. It seemed to me that being "in-love" was of the world while being love and loving was not. I just wanted to understand.

He explained to me that being in love was that first part of love; that part where you are so excited about seeing the person you adore and feeling his/her touch. Being in love was the butterfly feeling in your stomach, the joy in your mind that didn't allow you to sleep before you knew you would see each other again, and the anxiety that crept into your day when you were awaiting the next text from him or her.

It was the tears that were shed when you were parting at the airport and the longing that was felt when you wanted more time with each other. It was the part of choosing love with your romantic partner that wouldn't last. And many people who confused love with being in love didn't make it much farther than this; they confused being in love for love. They confused the butterfly feeling for the commitment.

"Some people are addicted to the being in love part." He added. "And they over-use the word love."

"What do you mean, they over-use the word love?" I asked completely clueless about what he meant by that.

"Well, it means that they say they 'love' ice cream when all they really mean is that that ice cream makes them feel good. So the 'in-love' part of love is the feel good part. The part that folks focus on when it feels good and happy and …"

"Warm fuzzies?' I interrupted, excited again to participate in the conversation.

Karl looked down at me; he towered over me at 6'4". The half-smile that was so classic to his demeanor made its way onto his face and his eyes smiled as well when they met mine. "Yes, he warmly replied. "And the warm fuzzies… the point is that most people use the word love when all they are referring to is a feel good feeling either toward people or toward food. The word has become disrespected in its over-use."

Karl's words landed heavily upon me as I recognized, in that moment, how often I personally over-used the word love. I used it to refer to ice-cream, peanut M&Ms, Diet Coke, red wine, walks on the beach, encounters with puppies…the list went on and on. He was right. I over-used the word love in these situations.

Karl's description interrupted my thoughts as he went onto explain that being love was something far beyond a feel good feeling. Being love was a commitment to well, being loving, and to being loving no matter what. Being loving no matter what didn't mean that you didn't call out another when their behavior was creating pain or when they were not taking responsibility for actions that were harmful to themselves or to others. It meant that above all else, you would love that person for what they are and what they are not. You would love them for who they are and who they are not. You would be love in all situations.

Yet, being loving, he emphasized did not mean that you would not hold the ones you loved accountable for their own authenticity or their own actions. A big part of being loving was being present for those you loved so they could rise to who they are and who they are becoming as defined by their own personal return to authenticity. It meant helping correct the ones you loved as they moved forward in their authenticity and it meant to receive their corrections as well. There was nothing passive about being loving. It wasn't for the weak of heart or those who lacked courage.

Karl further emphasized what I had come to realize through conversations with my friends. There was no room for jealousy in love. Being love was all about celebrating the other's greatness and facilitating them to their greatness but not managing them to become great. The difference, as I understood it, was that managing another in any form meant that manipulation was involved; that your actions and words were being motivated by self interest or the interest in a particular agenda versus the investment in knowing that the person you were involved in relationship was as holy as you, as god-like as you. And to be one in Christ, one in the Universe, to be truly connected meant that you were invested in facilitating them to their greatness just as much as you were invested in your own greatness and vice versa.

"Thank you Karl." I genuinely replied, grateful to him for his assistance. I understood what he was describing. Now, I just needed to know what being love in a romantic relationship looked like. I wanted to ask him but I refrained. I decided that it would be best for me to experience that myself it would be best for me to stop talking about it and move toward feeling it; toward feeling being in love and its movement to being love for myself. The question that seemed to remain was simply, was I ready to experience it? I decided I was.

I pulled down gently on Karl's hand just as we stepped closer to the barrier rocks on the Coronado beach.

Karl knew that was my non-verbal signal to him to make eye contact and he did. As he did, I gazed into his eyes. The warm butterfly feeling in my stomach returned and my groins grew warmer by the moment. He half-smiled again as our eyes connected and I reached my hand around to the back of his neck to pull him closer. His half-smile grew into a full smile as he bent his head toward mine. I stole a quick kind of friendship kiss, except for the fact that it was right smack on the lips. As our lips connected for the ever-so-brief moment, my whole face beamed with the kind of radiant joy that would compete with the sun.

Karl saw my radiating face as we pulled apart from the kiss and his smile widened. He looked out to the ocean and pulled me closer, holding me tight. The butterflies in my stomach were so active that I was confident my abdomen would take flight. My groins were so warm that it was all I could do to not wrap my legs around him right there and then on the public beach. He kept holding me tightly and I didn't want to ever let go.

"Karl," I finally spoke with the kind of thought that *I probably just ruined the moment with my words.*

"Hmm?" he responded with a gentle and soft rocking of his body.

"I love you." I spoke softly yet confidently.

"I know," he replied. "Thank you."

"And…" I hesitated a moment, checking in with my body, my soul, and my mind to see if I really wanted to go there. I did. "I am in love with you."

Karl stopped rocking me when I spoke those final words. My mind went into action with a retort to my mouth. *Oh shit. You did it now. You just fucked up this friendship. Why couldn't' you have just kept that comment to yourself?*

The other part of my mind retorted. *Hey, I am being authentic. This is how I feel and I checked in with you Ms. Smarty-Ass Mind. I checked in with you earlier and you didn't say not to say this. So quit blaming me. I said it, it feels right, honest and authentic, so shut up.*

I was so lost in my mind's dialogue that I had lost awareness of how Karl was responding to the announcement that I was in love with him.

Pulling me from the question of wondering how sane it was that my mind has conversations with itself, I felt Karl's hand softly touch me on my chin.

I looked up at him in response and the tears that were forming in my eyes clouded my vision. *Tears? Where did those come from? Was this a release of soul-felt emotion? Or did sand just blow up in my eyes?* Karl pulled my chin closer to his face. I smiled through the tears as I saw the smile on his face. He kissed me – it was a long, more than friend's kind of kiss, directly on the lips.

Yee-haw, I am in love!

CHAPTER TWENTY-THREE

Surrender

It finally came; a butterfly landed on my shoulder. I had just finished kayaking at Mammoth Lakes, California; it was my first time to this magical area. I was truly taken by the beauty of the place as well as the generosity of the people who had invited me to join them. They were loving, genuine, and authentic. They were taking care of me in a way that moved my soul. I was showing up in a manner of comfort and joy that I had never before felt among people that I had just met. I wasn't trying to mange any moment or any situation. I was just being present and feeling the love and the beauty all around me.

The butterfly, landing on my shoulder, signified to me a powerful transition – the transition to living in surrender. It was time for the transition to love fully, time to live in a state of being and in the present moment, to be open to that which comes next, to that which was right in front of me. I smiled at the butterfly, I thanked her for delivering her message, and I let her know that indeed I did know it was time…I am ready and all is well. I told the butterfly that the beauty of Her creation was right before me and my heart and soul were touched by it all. I told the butterfly that I surrender…to the truth. The truth that regardless of who I am or what I have journeyed through, life is indeed simple if I just choose to let go of all that keeps me from experiencing its joy.

The butterfly flitted for a moment around me and then kissed me on the cheek before returning to its perch on my shoulder; it felt like I had been kissed by truth. The truth… the truth either makes you laugh or it makes you cry. Either way, it moves you. In this moment, I was faced with the truth that the only thing these folks wanted from me was really…well…nothing. They were just providing a space for me to enjoy, to laugh, to love, to smile, to appreciate, to melt in with the beauty around me, and to shine with the magnificence of the mountains that surrounded us. The truth was that all I had to do was just be. And I accepted that offer in that moment. And in that moment of acceptance, the butterfly on my shoulder flew off to find another receiver of her message.

I stood on the bank of the lake upon which we had just kayaked. I felt as if I was an observer to all that was around me and I took a moment to retreat to a perch on a rock that looked inviting. I sat down in my quiet space and reflected upon the lessons I had learned in the past year. Edwardo had shown me that over-managing relationships not only creates stress for me, it creates stress for all those around me. He had taught me that just being with people as they figure out what they need in a relationship does not mean you are being used, it is an opportunity to practice listening to that which I desire and to practice being present in love for someone who is figuring out what they need. As the dream where I experienced the energy force attacking me reinforced, over-managing is pointless, life happens anyway. It is far more peaceful to choose how to receive it, to accept it, and to be with it, to learn from it and grow from it, rather than to try to negotiate it or manage it as it occurs. When I manage a situation, I miss the lesson I am to learn from just simply experiencing it.

I was grateful to Edwardo for remaining a friend to me, even though I pushed him away in my attempt to manage the outcome of our relationship. He was being love to me and I was grateful to him for role modeling that. As I glanced over to Karl from my perch on the rock, I saw his light Norwegian hair shimmering in the sun. It brought a smile to my face and in further gratitude, I reflected on the lesson that Ruben had taught me. He had shown me how to be both love and loving without fear and without worldly jealousy. He had shown me again what it looked like to be present and to just be in the moment while fully taking responsibility for one's own actions and recognizing how my choices could impact the joy of others.

Conversations with my friends had taught me about what it meant to be authentic – to show up as my true self, to show up consistently as who I was created to be and to explore with integrity "the me" I am becoming. My friends had taught me that being authentic in a relationship and being authentic in work were no different from each other. However, the conversations had also taught me that many times while at work, we choose to "park" our authenticity in order to manage another's ego by becoming what they need us to be in a moment or in something that is much longer than a moment. I had learned from these discussions and these conversations that if I don't recognize that I am parking my authenticity of if I leave my authenticity too long in the parking garage, the cost of getting my authenticity out of the garage is great; perhaps more than I can afford.

I had also learned from these discussions that I no longer wanted to show up as inauthentic in my personal relationship, especially the one I was enjoying with Karl. I was experiencing deep and profound joy in the freedom of being who I am and exploring who I am becoming with him. And I was also experiencing an expanding energy in the way we encouraged each other to shine our authentic lights in every situation. I felt no need to hide my greatness or its opposite with him and he was sharing the same feelings with me. It was pure unbounded ecstasy, like no other I had experienced thus far in my life. And I wished it for everyone I knew.

The sounds of a splash in the lake and a scream of excitement brought my attention from my reflections to a fish jumping away, free from a little boy's hook. I laughed as the father of the boy looked disappointed that the fish got away. The little boy on the other hand, looked full of joy. He didn't seem to care whether he had caught the fish or not. It reminded me of how grateful I was to have learned about the difference of inviting in experiences feeling responsible for what I created versus choosing the lessons learned from whatever flowed in and out of my life. The lessons learned by recognizing that the art of letting go was a moment-by-moment choice freed me from deep-seated feelings of guilt that in the past, I had invited in painful experiences for me and for others. I was young in my practice I knew, but just as the little boy was showing me, I could choose joy regardless of the outcome of any life experience.

I felt Karl's presence behind me. He had walked up to my perch as I was watching the little boy still smiling from the carefree experience of having lost a fish off his hook. As I turned slowly to see Karl's soft, gentle eyes, I felt a feeling that I had come to appreciate. Yet, it was a feeling that held no expectations. It was a feeling of being in love while being loving. The sight of Karl gave me the warm butterfly feeling while simultaneously providing me an opportunity to feel that my feet were planted firmly on the ground…rooted in a solid commitment of love.

Karl helped me realize that the love I was looking for all this time simply resided within me.

Karl helped me realize that I am love to anyone I choose to see as love and that they are love to me.

Karle helped me realize that I either receive that love or I do not. You either receive my love or you do not. When we both love and receive love, it reminds us of who we really are, which is perfect love, all of the time. All we have to do is accept where we are in the present moment of each moment, and let go of that which keeps us from fully surrendering to the truth that we are all god all of the time.

We choose to believe that which brings us peace. While what we believe may evolve or change over time, my prayer is that I choose to always believe in the sacredness of each one of us and the power that we have to choose to be love one moment at a time.

My prayer is that I continue to surrender to becoming my authentic self and to encouraging others to do the same.

My prayer is that each one of us surrenders to the love that we have deep within us; the love that resides and manifests itself apart from fear and the love that can indeed provide is with joy at the end of every outcome.

Hmmm…maybe I should explore more about how loving oneself, recognizing the dwelling place of the peaceful energy that resides within us all is a firm foundation upon which to build all relationships and all vocations. Yup, sounds like something fun; something to discover. I think I will record those lessons in something called, *The Foundation is Love.*

Namaste!

ABOUT THE AUTHOR

Marilee J. Bresciani is a professor of postsecondary education at San Diego State University. She has no expertise on the subject matter in this book, except that she has simply lived the life written about in this book and is still learning the lessons she shares. Her now more than twenty-four years of professional work has been committed to changing the way that America talks about quality of higher education. In order to keep from going crazy about trying to get the American public to care about what students are actually learning and how they are developing rather than other indicators that have nothing to do with that, she has sought out yoga and meditation. Marilee is currently undergoing yoga teacher training through the Baron Baptiste Power Yoga Institute. Marilee's mantra is "I teach what I need to learn."

More information about Marilee and her calling can be found at http://interwork.sdsu.edu/elip/consultation/wellbeing_yoga.html

REFERENCES

A Course in Miracles (ACIM) - www.acim.org

Baptiste, B. (2004). *40 Days to Personal Revolution: A Breakthrough Program to Radically Change Your Body and Awaken the Sacred Within Your Soul.* New York, NY: Fireside.

Baron Baptiste Power Yoga Institute – www.baronbaptiste.com

Bresciani, M.J. (2011). *Rushing to Yoga.* Bloomington, Indiana: Balboa Press.

Dyer, W. (2007). *Change Your Thoughts - Change Your Life: Living the Wisdom of the Tao.* Carlsbad, CA: Hay House Inc.

Gretzky, Wayne - http://www.brainyquote.com/quotes/authors/w/wayne_gretzky.html

Huddleston, P. (1996) *Prepare for Surgery, Heal Faster: A Guide Of Mind-Body Techniques.* Cambridge, MA: Angel River Press.

Lori Pettigrew, Astrologer, at loripettigrew@gmail.com

Menzel, Idina. *My Own Worst Enemy,* from the album "I Stand".

Merriam-Webster on-line dictionary; http://www.merriam-webster.com/dictionary/authentic

Nepo, M. (2011). *The Book of Awakening: Having the Life you Want by Being Present to the Life you Have.* San Francisco, CA.: Conari Press.

San Diego State University EdD Program Dissertation Information – http://interwork.sdsu.edu/eddleaders/community_college/program-requirements/dissertation.html

Thich Nhat Hanh, (1995). *Living Buddha, Living Christ.* New York, NY: Penguin Publishing.

Tipping, Colin. *Radical Forgiveness Steps* from – http://www.radicalforgiveness.com/

Virtue, Doreen (2004). *Archangel Oracle Cards.* Carlsbad, CA: HayHouse Publishing.

Walsch, N.D. (1997) *Meditations from Conversations with God.* Charlottesville, VA: Hampton Roads Publishing.

RESOURCES

- Phillip Urso – www.saltpondyoga.com
- Baron Baptiste – www.baronbaptise.com
- A Course In Miracles – www.acim.org
- The wonderful yoga instructors at Core Power Yoga in San Diego (www.corepoweryoga.com)
- Larger than life Lori Pettigrew, astrologer, at loripettigrew@gmail.com
- Dr. Charlie Sanders, Lifesource Network Chiropractic, at bodyheals@yahoo.com
- Dr. Adrian Bean at the Healing Point (www.thehealingpoint.com)
- Diana Pepper at Tree Frog Farm (www.treefrogfarm.com)
- Laura Lee, massage therapist (www.bikramyoga.com/studioDetails.php?id=278)
- Byron Katie's books (www.thework.com/index.php)
- Neale Donald Walsch, Conversations with God books (www.nealedonaldwalsch.com)
- Louise Hay's books (www.louisehay.com)
- Abraham Hicks's teachings (www.abraham-hicks.com/lawofattractionsource/index.php)
- Marianne Williamson's books (www.marianne.com)
- Deepak Chopra's books (www.chopra.com)
- Gary Renard's books (www.garyrenard.com)
- Thick Nhat Hanh books
- Core Power Yoga Studios, San Diego, CA (www.corepower.com)
- Amorah Kelly Acupuncture (www.amorahkelly.com)
- Chris Meredith – Psychic Medium – 760-743-5648

CPSIA information can be obtained at www.ICGtesting.com
Printed in the USA
LVOW110114120412

277219LV00001B/4/P